The Mind

Diet

Cookbook

Over 200 Mental Diet & Brain Health Recipes to Drastically Improve Brain Function & Have a Clear Mind. The Ultimate Guide to Prevent Alzheimer's, Dementia & Cognitive Decline. 14-Day meal plan included.

Author: Michelle Thomas

Special Bonus

Are you interested in receiving over 600 delicious recipes for FREE?

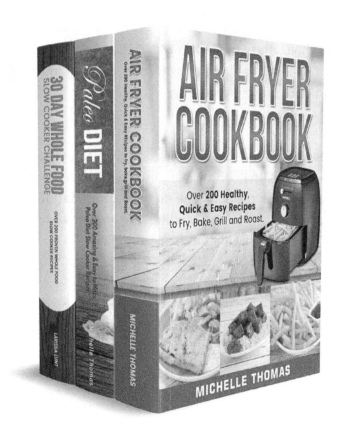

Only sign up for the cookbook box set if you are ready to be absolutely amazed with over 600 proven, delicious and easy to make recipes.

CLICK HERE or copy-paste www.bit.ly/2Ho82AH to get the free box set.

Happy cooking!

Description

Do you or a loved one suffer from a brain dysfunction like Alzheimer's Disease or Dementia? Did you know that the way you eat can significantly impact the onset or help regulate the related symptoms? That's right, a new hybrid diet has surfaced that has been proven to significantly aid in the improvement of brain functionality and help prevent or regulate a variety of brain diseases.

This diet is known as the MIND diet, and in this MIND Diet Cookbook, we are about to break the mould and not only introduce you to the diet by throw you right in the deep end with over 200 recipes to get you well on your way to recovery.

The acronym "MIND" was coined to explain a diet designed to prevent the loss of brain function and dementia as you age. The "MIND" initials are interpreted to mean Mediterranean-DASH Intervention for Neurodegenerative Delay. The diet is a combination of the DASH (Dietary Approaches to Stop Hypertension) the and Mediterranean diet which were designed to focus on a dietary pattern that supports your brain health and function.

This MIND Diet cookbook will provide a comprehensive overview of the MIND diet as well as explaining how to follow it. The Process is so thoroughly explained that even beginners can understand and follow the steps.

This MIND Diet Cookbook will explore:

- Over 200 Easy & Delicious Recipes for the MIND diet

- Access to Recipes that Include Detailed Nutritional Information, Ingredient List, Cook/Prep Time & Detailed Instructions

- Practical Guide to MIND Diet

- Top 10 Foods for Improving Cognitive Performance

- List of Foods You Must Avoid

- Lifestyle Guidelines for Optimal Brain Health

- Guide on Preventing Alzheimer's And Dementia

- Lunch Recipes

- Dinner Recipes

- Snack Recipes

- Dessert Recipes

- Mouth-watering Meat Recipes

- Easy Seafood Recipes

- Delicious Vegan & Vegetarian Recipes

- Amazing Soup Recipes

- Instant Pot Recipes

- Slow Cooker Recipes

- Dash Recipes for Two

Grab your copy of the MIND Diet Cookbook today!

Table of Contents

Introduction

The acronym "MIND" was coined to explain a diet designed to prevent the loss of brain function and dementia as you age. The "MIND" initials are interpreted to mean Mediterranean -DASH Intervention for Neurodegenerative Delay. The diet is a combination of the DASH (Dietary Approaches to Stop Hypertension) the and Mediterranean diet which were designed to focus on a dietary pattern that supports your brain health and function.

This book will provide a comprehensive overview of the MIND diet as well as explaining how to follow it. The Process is thoroughly explained, even beginners can understand and follow the steps.

What Is the MIND Diet?

Experts have reviewed the combination of the DASH and Mediterranean diets as a powerful and potent regime. Studies have revealed that these diets have positively impacted several chronic diseases including but not limited to lowered blood pressure, reduced risk of heart disease and diabetes.

To specifically target improved brain function and prevent dementia researchers created a diet for this purpose. To make this possible, they combined concepts from the Mediterranean and DASH diets that were proven to increase the brain's function.

This combined diet promotes the eating of berries because a direct correlation has been associated with improved brain functions. The individuals diet also recommends a high intake of fruits even though no link has been established with improved brain health. The MIND diet encourages the intake of berries but does not place any great emphasis on the intake of fruit in general.
No structured guideline on how to follow the MIND diet   has been established. However, the diet encourages the use of ten (10) specific foods and discourages the use of Five (5) in your everyday life.

The following section will discuss the foods to consume and avoid with the required servings for this diet.

Top 10 foods for improving cognitive performance
The MIND diet encourages the intake 10 following foods:

Beans:

This food should be Included in at least four meals per week. This diet recommends all beans, peas, lentils and soybeans.

Berries:
This food should be Included in at least two meals per week. Even though published research only refers to strawberries, other berries including blueberries, raspberries and blackberries should be incorporated for their antioxidant benefits.

Fish:
This food should be Included at least once per week. Try using fish that contains high amounts of omega-3 fatty acids like sardines, salmon, mackerel, trout and tuna.

Green leafy vegetables:
Try to consume at least 6 servings of green leafy vegetables weekly. This includes salads kale, spinach and cooked greens. Other vegetables types of vegetables should be used daily in addition to these vegetables. Non-starchy vegetables are more suitable because they contain a lot of nutrients and are low in calories.

Nuts:
Try to consume a minimum of 5 servings of nuts per week. A variety of nuts should be included.

Olive oil:
This food should be used as your main cooking oil.

Poultry:
This food should be included in at least twice per week. Fried chicken is not encouraged with this diet.

Whole grains:
This food should be included in at least three servings per day. Include whole grains like quinoa, oatmeal, brown rice, 100% whole-wheat bread and whole-wheat pasta.

Wine:
Both red and white wine can benefit the brain's health. However, most researchers focus on the resveratrol compound found in red wine, which can fight against Alzheimer's disease. Aim for no more than one glass day

Research has proven that even if the diet is not precisely followed you will still reap results. The MIND diet even in moderation is associated with a reduced risk of Alzheimer's disease. If you find yourself unable to consume the set amount of servings recommended, try not to quit the diet. You will get the best results from this diet if you stick to the recommended servings. Including more of the foods listed above has been associated with a lower risk of Alzheimer's disease, and better brain function over time.

Lifestyle guidelines for optimal brain health

Decreasing Inflammation & Oxidative Stress

Over the past couple of years many people have researched the MIND diet but has not been able to precisely pinpoint how exactly it works. However, it is believed by the scientists that created the MIND diet that by actively reducing the levels of inflammation and oxidative stress can significantly aid in achieving optimal brain health.

But what exactly is oxidative stress? This type of stress occurs when a large number of radicals or unstable molecules have accumulated in the body which in turn damages the cells. The cells in our brains are extremely vulnerable and as such fall suspect to damage whenever these radicals exist.

Inflammation, on the other hand, is a natural response of the body whenever there is a threat of infection or injury. IT is basically the body's protection mechanism. Though inflammation is useful in some cases, when the levels are not managed well it can become extremely harmful and aid in the creation of numerous chronic diseases.

When these two elements are combined they can form a severely detrimental weapon to our brains often resulting in cases of Dementia and Alzheimer's disease. As such by regulating or reducing the levels of inflammation and oxidative stress, it is believed that you can somewhat control or even prevent these diseases.

The foods we eat can greatly influence the levels of both inflammation and oxidative stress levels. It has even been found that particularly persons following the DASH diet and Mediterranean diets has been proven to have lower levels of inflammation and oxidative stress. This is actually what made the MIND diet so ideal for people trying to maintain great brain health. The MIND diet was created as a hybrid of both the DASH and Mediterranean diets, consisting of foods that all have anti-inflammatory and antioxidant effects.

Reducing Harmful Beta-Amyloid Proteins

Another benefit that the Mind diet is believed to give is the reduction of harmful beta-amyloid proteins in the brain. Like inflammation these beta-amyloids are typically present in the body, however, too much of it can be harmful as they accumulate and forms plaques in the brain. This is in no way a good thing as plaques can disrupt communication between cells and lead to the cells eventually dying. It is believed by many scientists that these plaques are the main contributing factor to Alzheimer's disease.

Studies done on Animal and test-tube demonstrates that the vitamins and antioxidants contained in many of the MIND diet foods may help in preventing beta-amyloid plaques from forming in the brain.

The MIND diet however, limits the consumption of foods which contain saturated and trans fats, which research has proven can increase the beta-amyloid protein levels in the brains of mice. Human observational research has found that the consumption of these fats led to a greater risk of Alzheimer's disease.

It is very important to note however, that this type of research is unable to elect cause and effect. Superior, controlled research is needed to determine exactly how the brain may benefit from the MIND diet.

List of Foods You Must Avoid/Limit

It is highly recommended by The MIND diet to limit the following foods:

- **Margarine and Butter:** You should try eating less than 1 tbsp. (roughly 14 grams) daily. Instead, use olive oil as your primary fat for cooking, and dip your bread if you must, in some olive oil laced with herbs.
- **Cheese:** The MIND diet highly recommends limited cheese consumption to once bi-weekly.
- **Red meat:** You should aim for no more than three servings weekly. This includes pork, all beef, lamb and by - products of these meats.
- **Fried food:** Absolutely no fried foods; The MIND diet totally discourages it, especially those from the fast-food outlets. Limit consumption to once bi-weekly or none at all.
- **Pastries and sweets:** This includes all the traditional desserts you can possibly think of; cookies, cakes, donuts, snacks, sweets and more also, majority processed junk food. These should be limited to not more than four times weekly. There are a variety of delicious MIND friendly desserts.

These foods contain saturated and trans fats hence Researchers discourage consumption of these foods.

Studies have shown that various types of diseases are associated with the consumption of trans fats. Heart disease and Alzheimer's disease are two of such.

Guide on preventing Alzheimer's and Dementia

The resistance of insulin and inflammation damage neurons and hinders communication among brain cells; this is what takes place in Alzheimer's disease. It is sometimes referred to as "diabetes of the brain." More than one research done demonstrates a powerful link betwixt metabolic disorders and the signal processing systems. If eating habits are adjusted, however, this can reduce inflammation and the brain protected.

Healthy Eating Tips

Reduce sugar intake. Refined carbohydrates such as pasta, white rice, white flour and sugary foods can and will lead to considerable spikes in your blood sugar which will eventually inflame your brain. Be careful of hidden sugar in packaged foods including cereals and bread, low fat or no fat products.

Enjoy a Mediterranean diet. Many epidemiological studies have shown that consuming a Mediterranean diet adequately lessens the risk of Alzheimer's and cognitive impairment. That means a restriction of processed foods; vegetables galore, fish, legumes, whole grains, and olive oil.

Avoid trans fats. These fats have the capacity to cause inflammation, and also create free radicals—these are both rigid on the brain. Consumption can be reduced by staying away from fast food, fried foods, packaged foods, also foods that includes "partially hydrogenated oils."

Get plenty of omega-3 fats. There is evidence that demonstrates the DHA that is found in these "fats" may aid in the prevention of dementia and Alzheimer's disease; being made possible by the reduction of beta-amyloid plaques. Food sources that contributes to this include tuna, mackerel, trout, salmon, sardines and seaweed. Fish oil can also be supplemented.

Stock up on fruit and vegetables. The more fruit and vegetables you eat, the better it is for you. In order to maximize protective vitamins and antioxidants, you have to eat across the color spectrum. These include, cruciferous vegetables (broccoli), green leafy vegetables and berries.

Enjoy daily cups of tea. Frequent consumption of magnificent tea may increase mental alertness and memory and will delay brain aging. Another brain healthy source is oolong and white teas. If you practise drinking up to 4 cups daily you will see increased benefits. Although coffee is not nearly as strong as tea, it also has brain benefits.

Cook at home often. Home cooked meals are the best. When you cook at home you can be sure your meals are fresh and wholesome; brain healthy nutrients are high and salt, sugar, additives and unhealthy fats are in low supply.

Supplements that may help prevent dementia

Magnesium, folic acid, vitamin D, vitamin B12, and fish oil may help in the preservation of brain health. Research demonstrates that vitamin E, ginkgo biloba, turmeric and coenzyme Q10 have yielded less convincing results; however, it may also aid in the prevention or delaying of dementia and Alzheimer's symptoms.

Always consult your medical practitioner before starting any diet.

A Sample Meal Plan for 14 Days

Whoever said that MIND diet meals had to be complicated was badly mistaken! Below we have put together a very simple and easy meal plan that is comprised of the 10 food groups generally recommended for the MIND diet to help you see how easy it is to avoid or limit the 5 forbidden foods.

What's even better is that every single meal added to this plan has been included in our recipe listing below so you should have no issues enjoying delicious MIND diet meals and staying on track.

Day 1
- **Breakfast:** Sweet Potato Oats Pie
- **Lunch:** Brussel Sprout and Apple Salad
- **Dinner:** Alfredo Spinach Lasagna

Day 2
- **Breakfast:** Cinnamon Apple Quinoa
- **Lunch:** Greek Style Chicken Wraps
- **Dinner:** BBQ Salmon with Sweet Potato

Day 3
- **Breakfast:** Egg Sandwich
- **Lunch:** Superfood Salmon Salad
- **Dinner:** Moroccan Flavored Duck Ragu

Day 4

- **Breakfast:** Cereal with Milk and Peaches
- **Lunch:** Chia-Crusted Chicken
- **Dinner:** Spicy Thai Peanut Noodles

Day 5

- **Breakfast:** Egg Sandwich
- **Lunch:** Superfood Salmon Salad
- **Dinner:** Moroccan Flavored Duck Ragu

Day 6

- **Breakfast:** Cereal with Milk and Peaches
- **Lunch:** Chia-Crusted Chicken
- **Dinner:** Spicy Thai Peanut Noodles

Day 7

- **Breakfast:** Sweet Potato Oats Pie
- **Lunch:** Brussel Sprout and Apple Salad
- **Dinner:** Alfredo Spinach Lasagna

Day 8

- **Breakfast:** Cinnamon Apple Quinoa
- **Lunch:** Greek Style Chicken Wraps
- **Dinner:** BBQ Salmon with Sweet Potato

Day 9

- **Breakfast:** Egg Sandwich
- **Lunch:** Superfood Salmon Salad
- **Dinner:** Moroccan Flavored Duck Ragu

Day 10

- **Breakfast:** Cereal with Milk and Peaches
- **Lunch:** Chia-Crusted Chicken
- **Dinner:** Spicy Thai Peanut Noodles

Day 11

- **Breakfast:** Sweet Potato Oats Pie
- **Lunch:** Brussel Sprout and Apple Salad
- **Dinner:** Alfredo Spinach Lasagna

Day 12

- **Breakfast:** Cinnamon Apple Quinoa

- **Lunch:** Greek Style Chicken Wraps
- **Dinner:** BBQ Salmon with Sweet Potato

Day 13
- **Breakfast:** Egg Sandwich
- **Lunch:** Superfood Salmon Salad
- **Dinner:** Moroccan Flavored Duck Ragu

Day 14
- **Breakfast:** Cereal with Milk and Peaches
- **Lunch:** Chia-Crusted Chicken
- **Dinner:** Spicy Thai Peanut Noodles

Tips for Following This Plan

- If you are a person who likes to enjoy the finer aspects of life, like a glass of wine then you will be pleased to know that enjoying a glass of wine with dinner on the MIND diet is actually recommended.
- If you find that you get the munchies between meals then nuts can be used as a quick snack.
- Try to make your own salad dressings at home with olive oil and other healthy ingredients to avoid hidden forbidden foods.

Mind Diet Breakfast Recipes

1. Muesli

Ingredients:

2 tbsp raisins

½ cup oats, raw

¼ cup apple, chopped

1 tbsp almonds (slivered), or 6 chopped almonds

2 oz milk, fat-free

4 oz plain yogurt, low-fat

½ tsp honey, if desired

Directions:

Mix together all the ingredients in a bowl. Serve immediately.

Serves: 1	**Prep Time:5 mins.**		**Cooking Time: 0 mins.**
Calories:361	**Protein:17g**	**Carbs:57g**	**Fat:8.5g**

2. Breakfast Quesadilla

Ingredients:

2 egg whites

1 egg

1 tsp olive oil

1 tortilla (whole wheat), 8-inch

4 oz orange juice or black currant juice

¼ cup salsa

2 tbsp plain yogurt, low-fat

Directions:

Pour olive oil in a nonstick skillet. Scramble the egg whites and eggs for a few minutes. Fill the tortilla with the eggs. Fold the tortilla in half. Heat in a skillet or microwave for about 1 minute per side. Top with salsa and yogurt. Serve with the orange juice or black currant juice.

Serves: 1	**Prep Time:5 mins.**		**Cooking Time:10 mins.**
Calories:352	**Protein:23g**	**Carbs:35g**	**Fat:15g**

3. Baked Eggs with Tomato and Spinach
Ingredients:

1 can (400g) tomatoes, chopped   4 eggs

1 bag (100g) spinach   1 tsp chili flakes

Directions:

Heat the oven to 200°C. Place spinach in a colander. Pour boiling water over the leaves to wilt them. Squeeze out the spinach's excess water and divide the vegetables among 4 small dishes (ovenproof).

Mix the tomatoes with some seasoning and the chili flakes. Add to the spinach. In each dish, make a well in the center, and crack open an egg. Bake for about 12 to 15 minutes. You may even bake the eggs longer, depending on your eggs' doneness. If desired, serve with crusty bread.

Serves: 4	**Prep Time:5 mins.**		**Cooking Time:15 mins.**
Calories:114	**Protein:9g**	**Carbs:3g**	**Fat:7g**

4. Lox Toast
Ingredients:

2 slices toast, whole wheat   1 tsp. mayonnaise

2 oz salmon, smoked   6 oz orange juice or 1 medium orange

2 slices red onion

Directions:

Top the toast with the mayonnaise, salmon, and onion. Serve with orange juice or orange. Enjoy.

Serves: 1	**Prep Time:5 mins.**		**Cooking Time: 0 mins.**
Calories:338	**Protein:24g**	**Carbs:52g**	**Fat:4.5g**

5. Waffle Parfait
Ingredients:

2 waffles, whole grain   2 tsp flaxseed, ground

½ cup yogurt (plain), low-fat   ½ cup berries (frozen), thawed

Directions:

Top the waffles with yogurt, flaxseed, and berries.

Serves: 1	**Prep Time:5 mins.**		**Cooking Time: 0 mins.**
Calories:367	**Protein:24g**	**Carbs:44g**	**Fat:11.5g**

6. Egg Sandwich

Ingredients:

1 tsp olive oil

1 egg

1 English muffin, whole wheat

3 baby spinach leaves

1 slice tomato

1 small apple

Directions:

In a skillet, fry the egg in olive oil. Fill the English muffin with tomato, fried egg, and spinach. Serve the sandwich with an apple on the side. Enjoy.

Serves: 1   **Prep Time:5 mins.**   **Cooking Time: 5 mins.**

Calories:360   **Protein:20g**   **Carbs:50g**   **Fat:12g**

7. Cereal with Milk and Peaches

Ingredients:

½ cup cereal, high-fiber

¾ cup cereal, whole grain

1 medium peach, sliced

4 tsp pumpkin seeds

8 oz milk, fat-free

Directions:

Mix together all the cereals. Top with the peach, pumpkin seeds, and milk. Serve and enjoy.

Serves: 1   **Prep Time:5 mins.**   **Cooking Time: 0 mins.**

Calories:348   **Protein:18g**   **Carbs:75g**   **Fat:6.5g**

8. Spinach Omelet

Ingredients:

1 bag (400g) spinach leaves

1 onion (large), sliced finely

3 tbsp olive oil

10 eggs

2 potatoes (large), peeled and sliced finely

Directions:

Place the spinach in a container. Boil a kettleful of water in a pot. Pour the water slowly over the spinach until it's wilted. Cool then under cold water. Squeeze out all the spinach's liquid and set the dried spinach aside. Place the grill to high heat. In a non-stick frying pan, heat the oil and cook gently the potato and onion for 10 minutes, or until the potato becomes soft. As the onion cooks, beat eggs in a large bowl and season with pepper and salt.

Add the spinach to the potatoes. Pour the eggs and cook until the eggs are almost set. Stir occasionally. Place omelet under grill to cook the top. Put the omelet on a plate, then turn over back to the frying pan. Continue to the cook the omelet on its underside and turn out on a chopping board. Cut to wedges. Serve hot.

Serves: 6	Prep Time:5 mins.		Cooking Time:10 mins.
Calories:209	Protein:12g	Carbs:11g	Fat:13g

9. Yogurt Parfait

Ingredients:

½ cup wheat squares, shredded

¾ cup yogurt (plain), low-fat

1 tbsp walnuts, chopped

¼ cup cereal, high-fiber

¼ cup berries

¼ banana, sliced

Directions:

In a bowl, layer the ingredients. Serve immediately.

Serves: 1	Prep Time:5 mins.		Cooking Time: 0 mins.
Calories:336	Protein:16g	Carbs:59g	Fat:9g

10. Superfood French Toast with Chia-Raspberry Jam and Yogurt

Ingredients:

Raspberry-chia jam:

½ cup fresh or frozen raspberries, if frozen, thaw before using

1 teaspoon maple syrup

2 teaspoons chia seeds

¼ cup plain, low fat Greek yogurt

French toast:

1 egg

2 tablespoons low-fat milk

½ teaspoon vanilla

Pinch of ground cinnamon

1 slice sprouted grain bread

1 teaspoon sunflower seed oil

Directions:

To make the raspberry-chia jam, put maple syrup and raspberries in a food processor or blender. Pulse until the mixture becomes smooth and evenly combined. Pour the jam into a bowl. Add the chia seeds. Stir until the seeds are evenly mixed throughout the jam. Set the jam aside. Place egg, milk, cinnamon and vanilla in a bowl. Whisk together until combined evenly. Dip bread into the egg mixture. Soak the bread until it is saturated with the egg mixture. Place a medium-sized skillet over a hot stove. Add the sunflower seed oil.

Wait until oil is hot before putting the bread on the skillet. Cook the soaked bread until the bottom starts to turn golden brown. Flip the bread to cook the other side. Cook until the toast is firm and both sides are golden brown. This will take around 6 minutes. Once toast is done, transfer to a plate. Spread a tablespoon of raspberry-chia jam over the toast. Top with some Greek yogurt.

Serves: 1	Prep Time:15 mins.		Cooking Time: 6 mins.
Calories:369	Protein:15g	Carbs:41g	Fat:15g

11. Oatmeal and Trail Mix Cupcakes

Ingredients:

1 1/4 cup mashed over-ripe banana

2.5 cups rolled oats

1/2 teaspoon salt

2 1/2 tablespoons pure honey, maple syrup, or agave

1/2 teaspoon cinnamon

2 tablespoon oat bran, flax meal or wheat germ

1/2 cup raisins, or dried cherries cranberries, chopped into smaller pieces

1 1/2 tablespoon oil

1 1/3 cup water

1 teaspoon pure vanilla extract

Directions:

Preheat the oven to 380 F. Place liners into 11 to 12 cupcake tins. Mix all the dry ingredients in a large deep bowl. Get another bowl. Place all the wet ingredients (liquids) inside this bowl. Whisk well. Carefully pour the wet ingredients into the dry. Stir until there are no visible dry ingredients. Divide the batter among the cupcake tins. Bake for 21 minutes. Broil the cupcakes for 3 more minutes to crisp up the tops. Set aside to cool.

Serves: 11-12   **Prep Time:15 mins.**   **Cooking Time:24 mins.**
Calories:98   **Protein:2.8g**   **Carbs:19.8g**   **Fat:1.3g**

12. Sweet Potato Oats Pie

Ingredients:

1 cup rolled oats

1 3/4 cups water

2-3 tablespoons brown sugar, maple syrup, or other sweetener of choice

1 sweet potato

1/2 tablespoon flaxseed meal

1/2 teaspoon ground cinnamon

3 tablespoons roasted pecans

Directions:

Set the oven to 400 F. Line a baking sheet with foil. Peel and slice the sweet potato in half. Drizzle olive oil, just enough to lightly coat the sweet potato halves. Arrange the oil-coated sweet potatoes on the prepared baking sheet; cut side facing up.

Roast the sweet potatoes in the oven for about 20 to 25 minutes, or until they are fork tender. Remove the roasted sweet potatoes from the oven. Set aside. Pour water into a saucepan. Allow to boil over medium-high heat. Add the oats slowly into the boiling water. Lower the heat setting to medium. Cook the oats according to the package instructions.

This can take about 5 minutes. Place the roasted sweet potatoes in a bowl and mash. Measure out about ½ cup of mashed sweet potatoes. Set aside in a separate bowl. Add the ½ cup of mashed sweet potatoes into the cooked oats. Fold in the flaxseeds, cinnamon and sweetener. Stir the mixture well.

If you want a thinner consistency, add a small amount of almond milk or other kinds of non-dairy milk. Ladle the oats into 2 serving bowls. Sprinkle with roasted pecans. Serve with a drizzle of honey if desired. Serve while still warm.

Serves: 2   **Prep Time:20 mins.**   **Cooking Time: 0 mins.**

Calories:253   **Protein:9.7g**   **Carbs:55.9g**   **Fat:8.8g**

13. Sweet Potato Waffles

Ingredients:

3 cups grated sweet potato
1/4 cup chopped spring onions, green part only
4 eggs, whisked
3 tablespoons coconut flour

1 teaspoon salt
1 teaspoon garlic powder
1/2 teaspoon ground black pepper
Coconut oil, for the waffle iron

Directions:

Squeeze the grated sweet potato to remove excess juice. Set aside in a medium-sized bowl. Put coconut flour, salt, pepper, garlic powder, eggs and spring onions into this same bowl. Stir the mixture to evenly distribute the ingredients. Heat up the waffle iron and coat the insides with a bit of coconut oil. Scoop out ¼ cup of the batter and gently pour it into the hot waffle iron. Cook the waffle. Serve the waffles while still warm.

Serves: 4   **Prep Time:10 mins.**   **Cooking Time: 5 mins.**
Calories:98   **Protein:4.2g**   **Carbs:14.6g**   **Fat:2.5g**

14. Artichoke Spinach Quiche Cup

Ingredients:

1 14.5-ounce can artichoke hearts, drained and chopped
1 package frozen spinach, thawed and drained
2/3 cup milk

5 eggs, lightly whisked
2 cloves garlic, minced
1/2 cup chopped white onion
1/4 teaspoon pepper
1/4 teaspoon salt

Directions:

Prepare the oven to 350F. Line 12 baking cups with cupcake liners. Place all the listed ingredients in a large mixing bowl. Stir into a well-combined batter. Scoop batter into prepared baking cups, filling each until nearly full. Bake the quiche. Check if the filling is done. Insert a toothpick in the center of the quiche and it should come out clean. Remove the quiche from the oven and serve while still hot.

Serves: 3   **Prep Time:15 mins.**   **Cooking Time:15 mins.**
Calories:325   **Protein:25g**   **Carbs:18g**   **Fat:16g**

15. Grapefruit with Honey and Banana

Ingredients:

2 cups red grapefruit sections

1 cup sliced banana

1 tablespoon honey

1 tablespoon freshly chopped mint

Directions:

Get ¼ cup of juice from the grapefruit. Place grapefruit sections in a bowl. Add the rest of the ingredients. Stir gently to coat all the ingredients with the juice. Cover the bowl with plastic wrap. Chill in the refrigerator for a few hours. Serve chilled.

Serves: 3   **Prep Time:15 mins.**   **Cooking Time: 0 mins.**

Calories:238   **Protein:14g**   **Carbs:34g**   **Fat:5g**

16. Cinnamon Apple Quinoa Bake

Ingredients:

1 cup uncooked quinoa

1/2 teaspoon nutmeg

1 1/2 teaspoons cinnamon

1/8 teaspoon ground cloves

1/4 cup raisins

2 apples, peeled, diced

2 cups vanilla soy milk

2 eggs

1/3 cup almonds, chopped

1/4 cup maple syrup

Directions:

Preheat the oven to 350F. Grease an 8-by-8 or 7-by-11 inches baking dish. Place uncooked quinoa in a mixing bowl. Add the spices. Mix everything well with a large spoon. Pour the mixture into the prepared baking dish. Spread into an even layer. Spread the raisins and apples over the quinoa mixture. Crack the eggs in a bowl. Add maple syrup and soy milk to the eggs. Whisk to mix. Pour the egg mixture over the quinoa. Give the mixture a light stir. Sprinkle chopped almonds over the entire dish. Put the casserole in the preheated oven and bake for about 1 hour. The casserole is done if the mixture has set and only a small liquid remains. Set the casserole aside to cool. Serve while warm with a few spoonsful of plain Greek yogurt.

Serves:6   **Prep Time:15 mins.**   **Cooking Time: 1 hr.**

Calories:269   **Protein:9g**   **Carbs:44.3g**   **Fat:7g**

17. Eggs and Chicken Rancheros

Ingredients:

8 ounces chicken

Olive oil cooking spray

1/4 teaspoon salt

4 eggs

1 cup cooked lentils

4 small whole-grain soft tortillas

4 tablespoons salsa, divided

Directions:

Place a cast iron skillet over a stove set to high heat. Place chickens on a shallow dish, and sprinkle salt on both sides. Lightly coat chicken with cooking oil spray. Place the chickens on the cast iron skillet and sear both sides. Lower the heat and continue cooking the chickens until your preferred level of done-ness. Transfer to a plate and let the meat rest.

Wipe the skillet and coat lightly with cooking spray. Add the eggs and cook over heat set to high. Cook the eggs sunny-side up. This takes about 3 minutes. Set aside on a plate. Toast the tortillas on a stove or in a toaster oven. Place tortillas on four serving plates. Spread ¼ cup of lentils and 1 tablespoon of salsa. Top with 1 egg. Slice the chicken thinly and divide between the tortillas and then fold them over. Serve immediately.

Serves: 4   **Prep Time:15 mins.**   **Cooking Time:3 mins.**

Calories:352   **Protein:30g**   **Carbs:35g**   **Fat:12g**

18. Roasted Superfood Vegetables Frittata Recipe

Ingredients:

3 medium red bell peppers, remove and
discard seeds, slice into quarters
Nonstick cooking spray
1 medium onion, sliced into 1/2-inch slices
4 cloves garlic, keep unpeeled
2 large zucchini, sliced into 3-1/2-inch strips

1 tablespoon olive oil
1 teaspoon salt
1/4 cup fresh parsley, chopped
4 eggs plus 6 egg whites
1/4 teaspoon cayenne pepper

Directions:

Prepare the oven to 425F. Arrange the oven racks so that one is at the lowest position and another is in the middle. Take 2 baking pans with shallow bottoms. Line with foil. Spray the surface lightly with cooking spray. Put garlic and bell pepper in one of the prepared baking pans. Place onions and zucchini in the other pan.

Spray the vegetables lightly with some of the cooking spray. Place the pan with the onions and zucchini on the lower oven rack. Place the other pan on the center oven rack. Roast the vegetables for 15 minutes. Remove the pans and change the positions on the oven. Place the pan with the onions-zucchini on the center rack and the other pan on the lower rack. Roast for another 10 minutes, until the vegetables are charred.

Remove the pans from the oven and set aside for 5 minutes. Lower the oven temperature to 350 F. Remove the skins from garlic and peppers. Chop everything coarsely. Put in a mixing bowl. Add ½ teaspoon salt and parsley. Mix. Lightly grease the bottom of a 9-inch round baking pan. Put eggs and egg whites in a mixing bowl, season with the remaining salt and the cayenne pepper, and then whisk thoroughly.

Pour the egg mixture over the vegetables. Pour the entire mixture into the prepared round pan. Bake in 350-degree oven for 45 to 50 minutes. Once the center has set, remove the frittata from the oven. Let the frittata rest for about 5 minutes so it can set. Slice and serve while still warm.

Serves: 6	Prep Time:20 mins.		Cooking Time: 1 hr. 15 mins.
Calories:139	Protein:11g	Carbs:8g	Fat:7g

19. Sweet Potato and Egg Skillet

Ingredients:

1 large sweet potato
4 large eggs

1/2 teaspoon smoked paprika (or any seasoning of your choice)
pinch of pepper and salt, to taste

Directions:

Set the broiler to high heat. Pierce the sweet potato all over with a fork. Broil until tender. Remove from broiler and cool slightly. Place one oven rack on the broiler's highest or second highest level. Once cooled, slice the sweet potatoes into thin ¼-inch rounds.

Lightly grease a skillet. Arrange the sweet potatoes in the skillet in a single flat layer. Beat the eggs and pour them evenly over the sweet potatoes. Sprinkle with pepper, salt and paprika. Place the entire skillet in the broiler and cook for 3 minutes until the top turns golden brown and the eggs have set. Serve while still hot.

Serves: 2   **Prep Time:10 mins.**   **Cooking Time: 13 mins.**
Calories:216   **Protein:16g**   **Carbs:13.1g**   **Fat:11.4g**

20. Spicy Scrambled Eggs

Ingredients:

6 eggs
1/4 cup milk
1 tablespoon olive oil
1/2 cup onion
1/2 cup diced bell pepper

2 garlic cloves, minced
1 tablespoon chopped coriander
1 teaspoon cumin seeds
1 teaspoon ground turmeric

Directions:

In a large frying pan or skillet, warm the olive oil. Sauté the onion, garlic and pepper in the oil until they start to wilt. While those vegetables are cooking, beat the eggs and the milk in a small bowl until combined. Add the coriander, cumin and turmeric to the frying pan and combine with the oil and vegetables. Cook for one minute. Pour the egg mixture into the pan and scramble the eggs, mixing the spices and vegetables into the eggs. Serve with a hint of salt and pepper.

Serves: 2   **Prep Time:15 mins.**   **Cooking Time: 4 mins.**
Calories:365   **Protein:28.9g**   **Carbs:10.7g**   **Fat:37g**

21.Pumpkin Walnut Pancakes

Ingredients

1/2 cup walnuts

1/2 cup almond flour

Coconut oil for cooking pancakes

1 Tbs chia seeds

1/8 tsp salt

2 tsp cinnamon

1/2 tsp ginger, ground

1/2 tsp nutmeg, ground

1/4 tsp baking soda

1/2 cup pumpkin puree

3 eggs

2 Tbs maple syrup

1/2 tsp vanilla extract

2 Tbs coconut flour

Directions

Chop walnuts. Heat a pancake griddle to medium, or 350 degrees. In a bowl combine all the dry ingredients in it. In a small bowl whisk all the wet ingredients. Add combine both the dry and wet ingredients in a large bowl. Whisk till it is fully mix. If there are any lumps in the batter just know that it is still fine. Use enough coconut oil to grease the center of your pan.

Pour about 1/4 cup full of batter in the pan and spread it into a pancake shape. Cook the batter on the first side for about 3–4 minutes, carefully flip on the other side and cook for another 1–2 minutes. Repeat the same step of cooking the batter but add more coconut oil in the pan if needed. Serve with any syrup along with slices of your favorite.

Serves: 4　　　　**Prep Time:45 mins.**　　　　**Cooking Time:6 mins.**

Calories:282　　　　**Protein:12.8g**　　**Carbs:12.6g**　　**Fat:21.2g**

22. Quinoa Pumpkin Muffins

Ingredients

Quinoa
1/3 cup chopped dates
1/3 cup walnuts
1 cup spelt flour or flour of your choice
1 egg
2 Tbs chia seeds
1/2 tsp cinnamon
1/4 tsp nutmeg

1/4 tsp cloves (optional)
1/2 tsp salt
1/2 tsp vanilla extract
1½ cups pumpkin puree
3 Tbs coconut oil
2 tsp baking powder
1–2 Tbs maple syrup (optional)

Directions

Cook quinoa according to package directions, enough to make 1/2 cup cooked grain. Chop dates and walnuts. Preheat oven to 350 degrees. Prep muffin tins with liners or oil. Combine all the ingredients in a mixing bowl; blend well. Pour batter evenly into muffin tins. Bake thirty to forty minutes, or until the muffins are cooked through. Allow to cool before enjoying.

Serves: 6	Prep Time:10 mins.		Cooking Time:40 mins.
Calories:410	Protein:15.4g	Carbs:34g	Fat:26.5g

23. Breakfast Burrito

Ingredients

10 eggs
1 bunch green onions
1 cup mushrooms
1/4 cup cilantro
2 cloves garlic
1 avocado
1 lime

2 Tbs olive oil
1/2-pound ground bison
1 tsp turmeric
1/2 tsp cumin
1/2 tsp Himalayan salt
1 tsp pepper
1/2 cup sour cream (optional)

Directions

Separate eggs; put whites in one bowl and yolks in another. Chop green onions, mushrooms, and cilantro. Peel and press or finely mince garlic. Peel and dice avocado. Slice lime into wedges. Stirring frequently, brown buffalo in oil over medium heat, crumbling meat as it cooks. Add in green onions, garlic, turmeric, and cumin. When the meat is mostly cooked, add mushrooms and continue to cook, stirring frequently, until they are soft.

Stir in egg yolks and cook until set. Meanwhile, whisk egg whites, season with salt and pepper. Pour a quarter of the mixture into a lightly oiled skillet or omelet pan. Cook very gently over low heat for about thirty seconds, then cover and cook for a minute more. Slide the egg white "tortillas" onto a plate. Roll egg mixture into the tortillas, garnish with avocado, parsley, and a squeeze of lime. Serve with a dollop of sour cream, if desired

Serves: 4   Prep Time:20 mins.   Cooking Time: 6 mins.
Calories:604   Protein:37.2g   Carbs:12.8g   Fat:45.6g

24. Egg Cups

Ingredients

1 yellow onion
3 cups shiitake mushrooms
2 leaves kale
2 cloves garlic
1 tsp turmeric
1/2 tsp dried thyme

1/2 tsp oregano
1 tsp salt
1 tsp freshly ground pepper
1 Tbs olive oil
10 eggs
1/2 cup nutritional yeast

Directions

Finely chop onion, mushrooms, and kale. Peel and press or mince garlic. In a large frying pan, sauté onion, garlic, turmeric, thyme, oregano, salt, and pepper and olive oil over medium heat until onions begin to soften and spices are fragrant. Add mushrooms and kale, and continue to cook, stirring frequently, until the kale is bright green. Distribute mushroom mixture to ten muffin tins. Crack an egg into each tin. Distribute nutritional yeast among the tins. Bake for twelve minutes at 400 degrees. Allow to set for a few minutes before serving. Enjoy!

Serves: 6	Prep Time:45 mins.		Cooking Time: 12 mins.
Calories:289	Protein:20.9g	Carbs:8.6g	Fat:18.6g

25. Mozzarella and Zucchini Frittata

Ingredients

1/2 red onion
1 zucchini
1/4-pound cremini mushrooms
7 large eggs, beaten
2/3 cup fresh mozzarella

1/2 cup fresh basil
2 Tbs extra virgin olive oil
1/2 tsp salt
1/4 tsp pepper
1 tsp turmeric

Directions

Slice the red onion thinly. Slice the mushroom and zucchini. Dice the mozzarella. Preheat oven to 350 degrees. Sauté mushrooms, zucchini and onion in oil until soft; transfer to shallow baking dish. Whisk turmeric, salt, pepper, and eggs; pour over zucchini mixture. Bake for about 3 minutes or until eggs. Sprinkle basil and mozzarella on top; return to oven. When eggs are done, remove from oven. Slice and enjoy!

Serves: 4	Prep Time:30 mins.		Cooking Time:3 mins.
Calories:244	Protein:13.9g	Carbs:25.3g	Fat:11.3g

26. Spinach and Egg Bites

Ingredients

1 cup spinach

2 cups shitake mushrooms

1/3 cup green onions

1 large clove garlic

1/2 cup uncooked millet

2 cups water

6 eggs

1 cup coconut milk

1/2 tsp salt

1/2 tsp pepper

1/2 cup nutritional yeast

1 tsp turmeric

Directions

Roughly chop spinach. Chop mushrooms and green onions. Peel and press garlic. Preheat the oven to 350 degrees F. Oil muffin tin or use liners if you prefer. Toast millet in a medium-sized pot over medium heat, stirring occasionally. Add water and salt, cover, and increase heat to boil. Reduce heat slightly and continue to cook until water is absorbed. In a medium bowl, whisk eggs, coconut milk, salt, pepper, turmeric, and garlic. Toss together with millet, spinach, mushrooms, and green onions; mix very well. Spoon into muffin cups; bake ten to twelve minutes, or until lightly firm to the touch. Sprinkle with nutritional yeast as soon as the egg bites come out of the oven; allow to cool slightly before serving.

Serves: 4   **Prep Time:45 mins.**   **Cooking Time:12 mins.**

Calories:412   **Protein:28.7g**   **Carbs:33.5g**   **Fat:18.1g**

27. Spinach Mushroom Frittata

Ingredients

1 Tbs cilantro, finely chopped

2 cups fresh spinach, chopped

3 medium red potatoes, thinly sliced

8 eggs

1/2 cup nutritional yeast

1/2 tsp turmeric

1/2 tsp salt

6 tsp extra virgin olive oil

2 tsp vegetable or chicken broth

1 large shallot, chopped

1½ cups shiitake mushrooms, chopped

Directions

Beat together turmeric, eggs, nutritional yeast and salt. Set it aside. Add broth with ¼ of your oil to a skillet on medium heat. Add shallot and stir until translucent. Add mushrooms and sauté for 3-5 minutes. Stir in cilantro and spinach and sauté two minutes more, then add to the egg mixture.

Heat the remaining oil in large skillet over medium heat. Spread red potatoes over the skillet bottom in one or two thin layers and cook five minutes over medium heat. Pour vegetable and egg mixture on top of your potatoes; reduce the heat to medium, and cover. Cook about twenty minutes, periodically checking to see if eggs are firm. When done, run rubber spatula around edge of frittata, cut in wedges, and serve.

Serves: 4   **Prep Time:45 mins.**   **Cooking Time:37 mins.**
Calories:412   **Protein:28.7g**   **Carbs:33.5g**   **Fat:18.1g**

28. Amaranth Pancakes

Ingredients

1/4-inch ginger root

2 tsp coconut oil

1 lemon

1 cup amaranth flour

1/2 cup arrowroot powder

1/2 cup almond meal

1 tsp ground cinnamon

1 tsp baking soda

1/4 tsp cloves

1 egg

2 Tbs blackstrap molasses

1/4 tsp salt

water as needed for consistency

Direction

Grate ginger root. Melt coconut oil. Juice lemon. Mix dry ingredients in a large bowl, using a wire whisk, until well combined. Reserve. In a separate bowl, using a wire whisk, beat egg until it is lemony in color. Stir in ginger root, lemon juice, coconut oil, and molasses; mix well. Make a well in the middle of the dry ingredients. Gently pour liquid into the well. Using a wooden spoon, go around the outside edge of the dry ingredients to gently pull the dry into the liquid. Mix like this as gently as you can, just until all the ingredients are wet but some bits of dry remain. Drop the batter onto a lightly oiled griddle or frying pan, heated to medium-high. When edges begin to bubble, flip and cook other side.

Serves: 2   **Prep Time:15 mins.**   **Cooking Time:10 mins.**

Calories:194   **Protein:6.3**   **Carbs:22.8**   **Fat:9.7**

Mind Diet Lunch Recipes

29. Spicy Tuna Rolls

Ingredients:

1/3 cup mayonnaise, low-fat

2 cans (5 to 6 oz each) tuna chunks (light), drained

1 tbsp Sriracha or hot sauce

2 cups brown rice (cooked), cooled

1 scallion, chopped

2 tbsp rice vinegar

3 cups watercress leaves

4 pcs 10" wraps, whole grain

1 avocado (ripe), sliced into 16 pieces

1 carrot (small), julienned

Soy sauce (reduced sodium), for dipping

Directions:

In a medium bowl, combine the mayonnaise, tuna, scallion, and Sriracha or hot sauce. In a small bowl, combine the vinegar and rice. Spread ¼ of the tuna mix over a whole wheat wrap. Top with ½ cup rice, 4 avocado slices, ¾ cup watercress, and ¼ of the carrots. Roll and cut the wrap in half or in quarters. Repeat the process with the rest of the wraps and filling. Serve with the soy sauce. If desired, you may add wasabi paste to the soy sauce.

Serves: 4	**Prep Time:** 25 mins.	**Cooking Time:** 0 mins.
Calories: 503	**Protein:** 18g **Carbs:** 71g	**Fat:** 17g

30. Chicken Kebabs

Ingredients:

400g chicken thigh (lean), cut to 1 1/2" cubes
½ tsp cayenne pepper
1 tsp cumin, ground
1 tbsp olive oil
1 tsp sweet paprika, smoked
140g couscous
24 cherry tomatoes

140g frozen peas
400ml vegetable stock, hot
1 pack coriander (small), chopped
1 carrot (large), coarsely grated
1 pack mint (small), chopped
2 tbsp olive oil, extra virgin
Juice of 1 lemon

Directions:

Soak 6 wood skewers for 30 minutes in water, in order to prevent burning of the wood while cooking. Place the cubed chicken in a bowl with olive oil and spices. Combine the ingredients until the chicken is coated with the spices and the oil. Thread a chicken cube on to a skewer, then thread a tomato.

Repeat the process until you get 4 chicken cubes and 4 tomatoes into a skewer. Meanwhile, place the couscous in a bowl. Add the vegetable stock and peas. Stir, cover with cling wrap and soak for about 5 minutes. Heat a griddle. When the couscous has absorbed the liquid, fluff up the grains gently with a fork. Stir in the herbs, carrot, olive oil, and lemon juice. Mix well, season the mix, and set it aside.

Put the skewers on to the griddle and grill for 5 to 6 minutes. Flip the skewers and cook for a further 5 to 6 minutes, until the tomatoes and meat are cooked through and charred. Serve the couscous together with the skewers.

Serves: 3   **Prep Time:20 mins.**   **Cooking Time: 20 mins.**
Calories:466   **Protein:28g**   **Carbs:35g**   **Fat:23g**

31. Chicken Burger

Ingredients:

¼ cup mayonnaise, low-fat
1 ½ tsp thyme (fresh), chopped finely and divided
1 tsp Dijon mustard
5 tbsp shallot (chopped finely), divided
1/3 cup ham, finely diced
1 lb ground chicken
¼ tsp pepper, freshly ground
¼ tsp salt
12 leaves spinach (large), with tough stems removed
8 small or 4 large pumpernickel bread slices (toasted), cut in half

Directions:

Preheat grill to medium-high setting. In a small bowl, mix together mustard, mayonnaise, ½ tsp thyme, and 1 tbsp shallot. Set aside. In a medium bowl, put in 4 tbsp shallots, 1 tsp thyme, ham, chicken, pepper, and salt. Combine gently but don't overmix. Form into 4 ¾" thick patties. Oil the rack of the grill. Grill the chicken burgers, and turn once, cooking 4 to 5 minutes each side. The cooking temperature should be 165°F. Assemble the burgers on the bread with spinach and the herb mayonnaise.

Serves: 4   **Prep Time:15 mins.**   **Cooking Time: 20 mins.**
Calories:350   **Protein:29g**   **Carbs:20g**   **Fat:17g**

32. Sardine Fettuccini

Ingredients:

8 oz fettuccini, whole wheat
4 tbsp olive oil (extra virgin), divided
4 cloves garlic, minced
¼ cup lemon juice
1 cup breadcrumbs (whole wheat), fresh
½ tsp salt
1 tsp pepper, freshly ground
½ cup fresh parsley, chopped
2 cans (3 to 4 oz) sardines in tomato sauce (skinless and boneless), flaked

Directions:

Boil pasta according to package directions or for 8 to 10 minutes. Drain the pasta. In a non-stick skillet on medium, heat 2 tbsp olive oil. Add the garlic and sauté it until sizzling and fragrant, but not browned, or for about 20 seconds. Transfer the oil and garlic into a large bowl. In a pan on medium, heat the rest of the olive oil. Add the breadcrumbs. Cook for 5 to 6 minutes, or until golden brown and crispy. Transfer the crumbs to a plate. In the garlic oil, whisk the lemon juice, salt, and pepper. Add the pasta, sardines, and parsley. Stir gently to combine. Sprinkle with the breadcrumbs and serve.

Serves: 4   **Prep Time:15 mins.**   **Cooking Time:15 mins.**
Calories:480   **Protein:23g**   **Carbs:53g**   **Fat:21g**

33. Tuna Mac and Faux Cheese

Ingredients:

3 cups (8 oz) rotini pasta, whole wheat

2 tbsp all-purpose flour

1 cup milk (nonfat), divided

1½ cup nutritional yeast

¼ tsp ancho chili powder, ground

¼ tsp pepper, freshly ground

¼ tsp salt

1 can (5 to 6 oz) tuna chunks (light), flaked and drained

1 can (10 oz) diced tomatoes with green chilies, drained

¼ cup blue corn tortilla chips, crumbled

Directions:

Preheat oven to 450°F. Cook the pasta according to package instructions. Drain and rinse the pasta. Meanwhile, whisk 2 tbsp milk and the flour in a bowl. In an ovenproof skillet on medium, heat the rest of the milk until steaming. Whisk gradually several tbsp of the hot milk into the flour-milk mixture. Whisk the mix back into the skillet. Cook on medium and constantly stir for 1 minute, or until the sauce is slightly thickened and smooth.

Remove from heat and add the nutritional yeast, salt, pepper, and chili powder. Add the pasta and tuna and coat them well with the sauce. Top with the tomatoes. Bake for 20 to 25 minutes, or until bubbling and hot. Garnish with the blue tortilla chips.

Serves: 1   **Prep Time:25 mins.**   **Cooking Time:20 mins.**

Calories:442   **Protein:33g**   **Carbs:55g**   **Fat:11g**

34. Chia-Crusted Chicken

Ingredients:

2 tablespoons almond meal
6 small pieces of chicken breast tenders
½ teaspoon salt
½ teaspoon ground black pepper
2 teaspoons Dijon mustard
2 eggs
2 tablespoons chia seeds
4 teaspoons olive oil
4 tablespoons unsweetened shredded coconut.

1 teaspoon honey
4 teaspoons lemon juice
¼ teaspoon garlic powder
¼ teaspoon turmeric
1 ½ cups shredded Brussel sprouts
½ cup sliced red onions
1 ½ cups shredded kale
More salt and pepper, according to preference

Directions:

Preheat the oven to 400F. In a shallow dish, mix the chicken breast tenders and almond meal. Season with ½ teaspoon each of ground black pepper and salt. Toss to coat the tenders evenly. Place eggs in a bowl. Add Dijon mustard and whisk together well. In another mixing bowl, mix the shredded coconut and chia seeds together.

Dip the chicken tenders into the egg mixture first, and then into the chia mixture. Arrange the coated chicken tenders on a shallow baking dish. Bake in the hot oven for 10 to 15 minutes until the tenders are cooked through. While the tenders are cooking, toss the salad together. Place the shredded kale and Brussels sprouts in a mixing bowl. Add the sliced red onions. Toss well. Serve chicken once done with the vegetable salad on the side.

Serves: 2	Prep Time:20 mins.		Cooking Time: 0 mins.
Calories:562	Protein:45g	Carbs:22g	Fat:33g

35. Ground Turkey and Sweet Potato Skillet

Ingredients:

2 tablespoons extra-virgin olive oil

1 teaspoon garlic clove, minced

1-pound extra-lean ground turkey

½ cup diced onions

1 ½ cup diced sweet potato

½ cup diced yellow pepper

Freshly ground black pepper

Salt

A pinch of red chili flakes

Fresh parsley, sliced for garnish

Directions:

Preheat the oven to 400 degrees F. Pour olive oil into a cast iron skillet set over a stove on medium high heat. Once the oil is hot, add garlic and ground turkey. Break up the ground meat to prevent clumps. Cook the meat for about 7 minutes, stirring occasionally, or until the ground turkey is golden brown. Add the yellow peppers and onions into the meat. Keep cooking until the onions turn golden brown. Add chili pepper and sweet potatoes.

Season with a small amount of ground pepper and salt. Give the mixture a quick stir and cover. Cook until everything is tender. When the sweet potatoes have softened add a sprinkle of parsley for garnish and serve immediately.

Serves: 4   **Prep Time:15 mins.**   **Cooking Time: 12 mins.**

Calories:247   **Protein:11.1g**   **Carbs:15.8g**   **Fat:15.8g**

36. Salmon Superfood Noodle Bowl

Ingredients:

1 6-ounce salmon fillet, remove the skin, slice fillet into 8 pieces

5 ounces asparagus, sliced into thirds

4 ounces whole-wheat spaghetti or soba buckwheat noodles

Cooking spray

1 tablespoon toasted sesame oil

1/4 teaspoon salt

Juice and zest of 1-2 limes

1/4 teaspoon black pepper

1/2 small avocado, sliced into bite-size pieces

4 ounces cucumber, keep the skin on, slice into medium pieces

Directions:

Boil some water in a deep pot and cook the noodles until al dente. Soba noodles cook for around 6 minutes while spaghetti cooks for about 8 minutes. Once noodles are done, strain them and set aside. Reserve the pasta water. In the same water where you cooked the pasta, put asparagus. Cook for about 2 minutes until it turns bright green and al dente.

Drain and rinse the asparagus under cold running water. Place a skillet or grill pan over a stove set to medium high heat. Spray cooking oil over the skillet or grill pan to grease it lightly. Once the skillet or pan is hot, place the salmon pieces. Cook salmon until done, about 2 to 3 minutes on each side. Transfer cooked salmon on a plate and set aside.

Pour lime juice and sesame oil into a small bowl. Add lime zest and season with pepper and salt. Whisk together to create vinaigrette. Place the noodles in a medium-sized serving plate. Add asparagus, avocados and cucumbers. Pour the vinaigrette all over. Toss to combine. Top with salmon and serve.

Serves: 2	Prep Time:15 mins.		Cooking Time: 20 mins.
Calories:492	Protein:29g	Carbs:47g	Fat:21.9g

37. Seared Chicken Thigh with Pepper & Celery Caponata

Ingredients:

140 g fresh spinach

200 g chicken thigh

For the caponata:

oil spray

1 red onion, sliced

2 garlic cloves, sliced into slivers

2 sticks of celery, sliced crosswise

1 400-g can chop tomato

1 orange pepper, seeds removed and discarded, pepper sliced into quarters

1 tablespoon caper

25 g (about 9 pieces) black pitted Kalamata olive, sliced in half

1 teaspoon balsamic vinegar

½ teaspoon dried oregano

Directions:

Lightly coat a wide, large non-stick skillet with cooking spray. Place over a stove set to medium high heat. Put the garlic and onions. Cover the skillet and cook the garlic and onions for 5 minutes. Stir halfway to brown them evenly.

Put the tomatoes into the skillet. Fill the can of the tomatoes with water and pour into the skillet as well. Stir and place the rest of the ingredients for the caponata. Cover and let the caponata simmer on low heat setting for 30 minutes. Take a small frying pan or griddle, heat over a stove set to high.

Sprinkle a generous amount of ground black pepper all over the chicken. Sear the chicken on both sides. This will take about 8 minutes to sear both sides or until no longer pink inside. Set another pan over low heat. Place the spinach and cover. Cook until the spinach leaves are wilted. Transfer to a plate. Divide the caponata between 2 serving plates. Arrange the spinach on top. Slice the chicken into strips and arrange them on top of the spinach. Serve immediately.

Serves: 4   Prep Time:20 mins.   Cooking Time: 41 mins.

Calories:289   Protein:27g   Carbs:19g   Fat:10g

38. Superfood Salmon Burgers

Ingredients:

4 skinless, boneless salmon fillets, slice into medium-sized chunks

thumb-size fresh piece ginger root, grated

2 tablespoon Thai red curry paste

1 teaspoon soy sauce

1 teaspoon vegetable oil

1 bunch coriander, picked leaves from half of the bunch, chop the other

Lemon, sliced into wedges, to serve

For the salad:

2 medium-sized carrots

1 teaspoon golden caster sugar

2 tablespoons white wine vinegar

Directions:

Put salmon in a food processor. Add soy, chopped coriander, ginger and paste. Pulse the mixture until ingredients are roughly minced. Transfer into a shallow dish. Divide the mixture into 4. Form each portion into burger patties. Heat oil in a frying pan set over high heat. Once oil and pan are hot, fry burgers for about 4 to 5 minutes a side. Slice cucumber and carrots into thin strips using a swivel peeler. Add sugar and vinegar to the vegetables strips. Mix until all the sugar dissolves. Add coriander leaves and toss. Put salad on a plate, divided between 4 serving plates. Place a small serving of rice on each plate and top with one burger.

Serves: 4   Prep Time:20 mins.   Cooking Time: 0 mins.

Calories:292   Protein:29g   Carbs:7g   Fat:17g

39. Salmon with Broad Bean Salad

Ingredients:

250 g broad beans, fresh or frozen, removed from the pods

300 g small new potatoes, sliced in half

200 g tub roasted artichoke hearts in oil, drain but reserve its oil

4 spring onions, trim then slice

2-3 tablespoons extra virgin olive oil

1-2 preserved small lemons, use zest only, sliced finely

Salt

Black pepper, freshly ground

2 raw lightly smoked salmon fillets

Handful of fresh mint leaves, sliced into thin slivers

100 g wild rocket

1 lemon, sliced into wedges, to use when serving

Directions:

Boil water in a large pot and cook the potatoes for 10 minutes, or until fork tender. Put the beans into this same pot. Cook until just tender. Drain the vegetables. Rinse with running cold water to stop further cooking. Put potatoes in a large bowl. Pour in the oil reserved from the artichokes. Stir to coat the potatoes.

Add more olive oil as necessary. Set aside to continue cooling. Once cooled, place potatoes in a serving plate. Remove the skins from the beans and place in a bowl. Place artichokes pieces into the bowl with the beans. Put in sliced preserved lemons, remaining olive oil, seasoning and spring onions. Toss to mix. Place a small pan on a stove set to medium high heat.

Once pan is hot, cook the fish, skin-side down first. Cook for 3 minutes then flip to cook the other side. Lower the heat and cover the pan to finish cooking the fish. Turn the heat off. Let the fish cool slightly before handling. Remove the skin from the fish. Flake the fish and remove any bones. Add into the bowl with the beans. Add rocket and mint. Toss and spoon over the potatoes. Serve with some lemon.

Serves: 4   **Prep Time:15 mins.**   **Cooking Time:16 mins.**

Calories:311   **Protein:14g**   **Carbs:34g**   **Fat:16g**

40. Greek Style Chicken Wraps

Ingredients:

3 tablespoons coarsely chopped pitted Kalamata olives

1 cup halved grape tomatoes

1 tablespoon chopped fresh oregano

1 1/2 tablespoons fresh lemon juice

1/8 teaspoon ground red pepper

1 tablespoon olive oil

2 small or Kirby cucumbers, chopped

1 cup shredded boneless, skinless rotisserie chicken breast

6 pieces 8-inch whole-wheat flour tortillas

6 tablespoons plain hummus

Directions:

Toss feta, chicken, cucumber, pepper, oregano, olives, tomatoes, oil and juice in a large mixing bowl. Scoop 1 tablespoon of hummus over each tortilla. Spread all over. Scoop ½ cup of chicken mixture over one side of the tortilla's surface. Carefully roll the tortilla and slice each wrap in half.

Serves: 6   **Prep Time:20 mins.**   **Cooking Time: 0 mins.**

Calories:237   **Protein:12g**   **Carbs:27g**   **Fat:10g**

41. Roasted Red Pepper Greek Wraps

Ingredients:

1 10" whole grain wrap

1/4 cup sliced baby Bella mushrooms

1/2 cup baby spinach

1/4 cup roasted red pepper, sliced

1/4 cup sliced cucumber

1 tablespoon chopped green onions

2 tablespoons sliced olives

Directions:

Coat a skillet lightly with cooking spray. Set it over a stove on medium heat. Put the wrap on the hot skillet. Sprinkle the green onions, roasted red peppers and sliced mushrooms on top of the wrap. Let the wrap heat up and turn lightly brown. Transfer the wrap on a plate. Sprinkle the wrap with the olives, cucumber and spinach. Slice into half and serve with hummus if desired.

Serves: 1   **Prep Time:15 mins.**   **Cooking Time: 0 mins.**

Calories:236   **Protein:9g**   **Carbs:27g**   **Fat:13g**

42. Swiss Chard Wrap with Almond-Lime Dip

Ingredients:

Wrap:

1 peeled large beet, grated

2 peeled carrots, grated

1/4 teaspoon sea salt, divided

1 teaspoon extra-virgin olive oil

1/4 cup fresh cilantro leaves, chopped

2 peeled avocados, pitted then chopped

3 tablespoons fresh lime juice

1/4 teaspoon fresh ground black pepper

2 bunches Swiss chard

1 packed cup pea shoots or sprouts like broccoli, radish or alfalfa)

Sauce:

1/4 cup unsalted natural almond butter

2 tablespoons fresh lime juice

2 tablespoons raw honey

2 teaspoons reduced-sodium tamari

Directions:

Put all the ingredients for the sauce in a small mixing bowl. Whisk everything to combine into a smooth mixture. Set aside for later use. Get a medium-sized deep bowl. Put in beets, 1/8 teaspoon of salt, oil and carrots. Toss lightly. Get another medium-sized deep bowl. Put in cilantro, pepper, remaining 1/8 teaspoon salt, lime juice and avocados.

Stir and mash everything into a chunky mixture. Remove the spine from the chard leaves without splitting the leaf. Place leaves in a steamer basket and set over a large saucepan with about 1 inch deep of simmering water. Cover the steamer and cook the leaves until tender, about 3 to 4 minutes.

Remove the cooked chard and transfer into a plate lined with paper towels. Drain the excess water from the leaves. Assemble the wrap by scooping 2 tablespoons of carrot mixture into each leaf, at the stem side. Top with 1 tablespoon of pea shoots then a rounded 1 tablespoon of avocado mixture. Carefully roll the leaf, tucking the sides for a compact wrap. Serve immediately with the prepared dip.

Serves: 4	Prep Time:20 mins.		Cooking Time: 4 mins.
Calories:364	Protein:9g	Carbs:34g	Fat:25g

43. Sesame-Crusted Seared Salmon

Ingredients:

150 g brown rice noodles

2 100-g fillets of salmon, skin on

2 limes

4 teaspoon sesame seeds

4 teaspoons tahini

1 clove of garlic

1 ripe avocado

1 small cucumber

2 raw baby beets

2 small carrots

1 punnet cress

extra virgin olive oil

2 sprigs of fresh coriander

1 fresh red chili

Directions:

Cook the noodles according to the package directions and then drain. Sprinkle lime juice over the noodles and toss. Set aside. Slice each salmon fillet into 3 lengthwise sections. Place sesame seeds on a shallow dish. Coat one side of the salmon with sesame seeds by lightly pressing down into the seeds. Heat a non-stick pan on a stove set to medium heat. Once pan is hot, place the salmon with the sesame-crusted side down on the frying pan.

Cook until golden then flip to cook the other side. Transfer salmon to a plate. Put garlic and a pinch of salt in a pestle-and-mortar. Pound garlic into a paste. Add the tahini to the paste and muddle. Add a splash of water and lime juice to the garlic mixture the stir until smooth. Grate the beets, carrots and cucumber separately. Divide each into 2 piles, one for each serving plate.

Top the vegetables with cress. Divide the noodles between the plates. Arrange into a neat pile. Slice and peel the avocado. Remove the pit. Place half avocado in each plate. Carefully pour the dressing into the avocado well, where the seed used to be. Place salmon on each plate. Scatter coriander leaves over everything and serve.

Serves: 2	**Prep Time:20 mins.**	**Cooking Time: 0 mins.**
Calories:552	**Protein:28.4g**	**Carbs:35.1g**	**Fat:33.1g**

44. Super Bowl Honey and Turmeric Wings

Ingredients:

2 pounds chicken wings

1/8 teaspoon salt

1 tablespoon soy sauce

1/8 teaspoon chili powder

1 tablespoon honey

1/8 teaspoon ground turmeric

2 inches fresh, peeled ginger root

Directions:

Grind the ginger root in a small food processor or hand grind with a mortar and pestle. Extract the juice and discard the root. Marinate the wings with the seasonings and ginger root extract for 1-2 hours and bake or grill at 375 degrees for 25 minutes

Serves: 2	Prep Time:15 mins.		Cooking Time:25 mins.
Calories:314	Protein:50.2	Carbs:5.4	Fat:8.8

45. Chicken and Veggie Kabob

Ingredients:

1-pound chicken thigh, cut into cubes

1-pint cherry tomatoes

3 zucchini, cut into cubes

1 tablespoon ground turmeric

1 tablespoon ground paprika

1 tablespoon ground cumin

2 tablespoons olive oil

2 tablespoons red wine vinegar

Skewers

Directions:

Heat the grill and arrange the chicken, tomatoes and zucchini on skewers. Lay them in a baking dish. In a separate bowl, combine the oil, vinegar and spices. Pour it over the kabobs and allow them to marinate while the grill heats. Once you're ready to cook, lay the kabobs on the grill and cook until the meat is done, about 10-12 minutes.

Serves: 4	Prep Time:15 mins.		Cooking Time:12 mins.
Calories:314	Protein:50.2	Carbs:5.4	Fat:8.8

46. Beer Glazed Turmeric Bratwurst

Ingredients:

½ teaspoon of turmeric

1/8 cup Worcestershire sauce

1 12-ounce can of beer, any variety

1 teaspoon garlic powder

1-pound bratwurst

1 large onion, sliced and cut into half rings

Directions:

Combine all ingredients in a large skillet and bring to boil, then reduce heat and simmer for 20 minutes, turning occasionally. Drain. Cook bratwursts in the drained skillet until browned, turning frequently, or if desired, they can be finished on the grill. Scrape onions out to use as garnish.

Serves: 4	Prep Time:15 mins.		Cooking Time:12 mins.
Calories:552	Protein:21.2	Carbs:11.3	Fat:46.2

47. Festival Chicken Stir-Fry

Ingredients

1 shallot, finely chopped

2 cups shiitake mushrooms, chopped

3 large carrots, thinly sliced

6 cloves garlic, finely chopped

1½-inch piece ginger, grated

2 cups chicken, cooked, roughly chopped

1 lime, cut into wedges

2 Tbs coconut oil

1/2 cup coconut aminos

1/2 tsp Himalayan salt

1 Tbs turmeric

1/2 cup sugar snap peas

Quinoa, 2 cups, cooked

2 cups broccoli florets, chopped

Directions

In a large wok, heat the coconut oil. Add the mushroom and shallots then cook for 3 minutes. Stir often. Add carrots, broccoli, garlic and ginger; cook for 3 minutes, stirring often. Stir in turmeric, salt and coconut aminos. Add peas and chicken then cook until the chicken has been warmed through. Serve over quinoa and garnish with lime wedges.

Serves: 4	Prep Time:45 mins.		Cooking Time:8 mins.
Calories:217	Protein:21.6g	Carbs:13.4g	Fat:10.1g

48. Ginger Turkey Cutlets

Ingredients

1 bunch green onions
2 bulbs fennel
1/4-pound shiitake mushrooms
1 bunch chard
2 cloves garlic
2 inches fresh ginger
2 inches fresh ginger
2 limes
2 tsp toasted sesame oil
2 Tbs tamari
2 Tbs freshly ground black pepper
2 pounds turkey cutlets
2¼ cups chicken broth

1 can coconut milk
2 cups uncooked sprouted rice
1/2 tsp salt
4 Tbs coconut flour
2 Tbs coconut oil
3 Tbs tamari
3 Tbs rice vinegar
1½ Tbs red wine vinegar
3 Tbs maple syrup
3 Tbs almond butter
2 Tbs coconut oil
¼ cup chicken broth

Directions

Roughly chop onions, fennel, mushrooms, and chard. Peel and mince or press garlic. Grate ginger. Grate ginger. Juice limes. In a small bowl, whisk together sesame oil, ginger, tamari, lime juice, and pepper. Marinate turkey in this mixture for one hour. Meanwhile, start rice; bring 2¼ cups chicken broth and one can coconut milk to a boil over medium-high heat. Stir in rice and ½ teaspoon salt; cover and reduce heat to low. Simmer twenty minutes or until rice is tender. Remove from heat; set aside. When the marinating hour is nearly up, preheat oven to 350 degrees. Oil a large, ovenproof skillet, and heat over medium-high heat. Remove turkey from marinade, discard marinade.

Dust with coconut flour, and fry about one minute on each side. Cover and bake until turkey reaches an internal temperature of 170 degrees, or about ten to fifteen minutes. Remove from pan and set aside. For the sauce, whisk together fresh ginger, tamari, rice vinegar, red wine vinegar, maple syrup, almond butter, and 2 tablespoons water. Set aside. Sauté green onions and garlic in coconut oil over medium heat. Add fennel and mushrooms; continue to cook, stirring frequently until mushrooms soften. Add broth and chard and cook until bright green. Toss veggies with some of the sauce. Serve veggies and turkey over rice, with a drizzle of sauce.

Serves: 4	Prep Time:45 mins.	Cooking Time:37 mins.
Calories:459	Protein:44.2g	Carbs:29.7.4g	Fat:23g

49. Dandelion Greens Enchiladas

Ingredients

1 whole roasted chicken
2 bunches green onions
1 bunch dandelion greens
1/4-pound portabella mushrooms
6 cloves garlic

2 Tbs olive oil
1 cup chicken broth
1 package tortillas
1 (13-oz) jar green chilis or green chili sauce (including liquid)

Directions

Debone chicken, tear meat into bite-sized pieces, and set aside. Finely chop green onions, dandelion greens, and mushrooms. Press or mince garlic. Preheat oven to 350 degrees. In a soup pot, sauté green onions and garlic in olive oil until onions are soft. Add greens and mushrooms, and sauté until greens are tender and bright green. Add chicken, broth, and chili. Simmer for ten minutes. In a 9 x 13 baking dish, layer greens and mushroom mix with tortillas until dish is full. Bake for about 25 minutes.

Serves: 6	**Prep Time:15 mins.**	**Cooking Time:25 mins.**
Calories:705	**Protein:48.3g**	**Carbs:64.9g**	**Fat:26.8g**

50. Salmon and Sweet Potato Cakes

Ingredients

2 large sweet potatoes
1 shallot
1/3 cup parsley
1 tsp fresh rosemary
1 bunch green onion
2 lemons

2 6-oz. cans wild Alaskan salmon
1/2 cup cornmeal
1/4 tsp salt
3 eggs
3 Tbs extra virgin olive oil
4 cups mixed baby greens

Directions

Leaving skins on, cube sweet potatoes. Finely chop shallots, parsley, rosemary, and green onions. Cut lemons into wedges. Boil sweet potatoes for fifteen minutes or until tender. Drain and mash in large bowl. Add drained salmon, shallot, parsley, rosemary, green onions, cornmeal, salt, and eggs. Mix well. Shape mixture into palm-sized patties (about 2 inches in diameter). In large skillet, preferably iron, heat oil over medium-low heat. Add patties and cook until undersides are slightly golden (about three minutes per side). Use wide spatula to flip patties. Serve salmon cakes over bed of greens with lemon wedges.

Serves: 4	**Prep Time:15 mins.**	**Cooking Time:21 mins.**
Calories:423	**Protein: 28.6g**	**Carbs:37g**	**Fat:17.4g**

51. Turmeric Chicken and Brussels Sprouts

Ingredients

1-pound brussels sprouts
1 sweet potato
4 small shallots
1 lemon
2 sprigs rosemary
2 cloves garlic
4 Tbs extra virgin olive oil

1 tsp salt
1/2 tsp ground pepper
1 tsp cumin
2 Tbs turmeric
1 tsp dried thyme
2½ pounds chicken thighs

Directions

Preheat oven to 350 degrees. Trim and quarter brussels sprouts. Dice sweet potatoes. Peel and quarter shallots. Slice lemon into thin pinwheels. Stem rosemary, and finely chop leaves. Peel and mince garlic. Combine brussels sprouts, sweet potato, shallots, lemon, 2 tablespoons oil, 1/4 teaspoon pepper, 1/2 teaspoon salt, and cumin in a large baking dish. Mash garlic and the remaining 1/2 teaspoon salt with side of a knife to form a paste. Combine with rosemary, turmeric, thyme, remaining 1/4 teaspoon pepper, and remaining 2 tablespoon oil. Rub paste over chicken. Nestle chicken in with brussels sprouts and sweet potato. Roast, lightly covered with foil, until done, about twenty minutes for bone-in, and ten to twelve minutes for boneless. Serve chicken with brussels sprouts and sweet potato.

Serves: 4   **Prep Time:45 mins.**   **Cooking Time:21 mins.**
Calories:423   **Protein: 28.6g**   **Carbs:37g**   **Fat:17.4g**

52.Sweet Potato Chard Wraps

Ingredients

1 large shallot, finely chopped

2 cloves of garlic, finely chopped

1 lime, juiced

1 can black beans, or 2 cups cooked beans, rinsed and drained

1 large sweet potato, grated

1 bunch chard, leaves removed, stems chopped finely

1 avocado, peeled, pitted

1/4 cup cilantro, chopped

1 Tbs coconut oil

2 tsp curry powder

1/2 tsp turmeric

2 tsp cumin

1/2 tsp chili powder (optional)

Salt and pepper to taste

1/2 cup water

Directions

Sauté garlic and shallot in coconut oil until shallot becomes translucent. Add in spices, and sauté for a bit longer, while stirring. Add water, lime juice, water, chard stems, and sweet potatoes; cover and simmer until sweet potatoes are almost cooked, stir occasionally and watch to see if more water is needed. Add beans then continue cooking until beans the liquid fully cooks out. Rinse chard leaves, but don't dry them. Set a skillet over medium heat then add leaves, and cover. Allow to steam with the water from rinsing the leaves (about 1 minute). Wrap a few spoonful of the filling in each leaf. Garnish with cilantro and avocado.

Serves: 4   Prep Time:15 mins.   Cooking Time:20 mins.

Calories:170   Protein:2.7g   Carbs:17.6g   Fat:11.3g

53. Crab Cakes

Ingredients

1 egg, lightly beaten
1/2 c chopped green onions
2 Tbs mayonnaise
1 Tbs cilantro, chopped
16 oz crab meat
1 Tbs Old Bay seasoning
1/3 tsp turmeric
1/4 tsp pepper

1/2 c extra virgin olive oil
3 Tbs fresh squeezed lemon juice
1 tsp brown mustard
1 clove fresh garlic, crushed
1 tsp raw honey
1 lemon, cut into wedges
Fresh mixed greens of your choice

Directions

Preheat oven to 350 degrees. Line a baking sheet with parchment paper. Begin by preparing crab cakes. In a large bowl, combine lightly beaten egg, onions, mayonnaise, cilantro, crab meat, Old Bay seasoning, turmeric, and pepper. Mix well and form into patties. Arrange on baking sheet and sprinkle with additional Old Bay. Bake 25 minutes, or until cooked through. Honey Mustard Vinaigrette While crab cakes are baking, make vinaigrette. In a small bowl, combine extra virgin olive oil, lemon juice, mustard, garlic, and honey. Whisk until well-combined and refrigerate until ready to serve. Serve on a bed of mixed greens with a squeeze of lemon and a drizzle of vinaigrette.

Serves: 4   Prep Time:15 mins.   Cooking Time:25 mins.
Calories:170   Protein:2.7g   Carbs:17.6g   Fat:11.3g

54.Jicama Lettuce Wraps

Ingredients

1/4 cup pumpkin seeds

1 Tbs fresh mint

1 bunch parsley

1 bunch radishes

1/2-pound jicama

2 carrots

1 cucumber

1 large avocado

8 kalamata olives

1/2 lemon

1/4 cup extra virgin olive oil

2 Tbs apple cider vinegar

1/2 tsp Himalayan sea salt

1 tsp cumin

1/2 tsp ground black pepper

Romaine or another lettuce

Directions

Toast pumpkin seeds in a dry skillet over medium heat, stirring occasionally. Finely chop mint, parsley, and radishes. Peel and finely chop jicama. Seed and dice cucumber. Peel, pit, and dice avocado. Pit and mince olives. Juice lemon. In a small bowl, whisk together olive oil, vinegar, lemon juice, and salt. Combine pumpkin seeds, cumin, veggies, olives, and mint in a large bowl; mix well. Toss with dressing. Let sit fifteen minutes or more before serving. Spoon jicama mixture into lettuce leaves and roll.

Serves: 4   **Prep Time:35 mins.**   **Cooking Time:0 mins.**

Calories:289   **Protein:5.1g**   **Carbs:27.4g**   **Fat:19.3g**

55.Zesty Chicken Patties

Ingredients

2 garlic cloves, finely chopped

2/3 cup cilantro, chopped

3 green onions, chopped

1 tsp fresh ginger, grated

1-pound ground chicken

1 tsp red chili powder (or to taste)

1 tsp fish sauce

½ tsp Himalayan salt

½ tsp pepper

½ lime

½ tsp turmeric

2 Tbs coconut oil

2 Tbs hemp seeds

Mixed salad greens for serving

Directions

Mix turmeric, lime juice, pepper, salt, fish sauce, chili, ginger, onions, cilantro and chicken. Use the mixture to form patties then lightly rub with oil. Roll the edges in hemp seeds and sauté until cooked (about 8 minutes per side). Serve over greens.

Serves: 4   **Prep Time:15 mins.**   **Cooking Time:20 mins.**

Calories:338   **Protein:22.5g**   **Carbs:3.2g**   **Fat:26.3g**

56. Mediterranean Turkey Patties

Ingredients

1/2 cup shallots	1 cup plain Greek yogurt
3 cloves garlic	1/2 tsp Himalayan salt
2 tsp fresh thyme	1/2 tsp turmeric
1 Tbs fresh basil	1/2 tsp pepper
3 leaves chard	1/2 tsp Himalayan salt
1 lemon	1-pound ground turkey meat
1 Tbs mint leaves	1 Tbs hemp hearts
1 Tbs chives	2 Tbs coconut oil
1 bunch green onions	2 cups mixed greens
1 cucumber	

Directions

Blend in a food processor, or use a knife to finely chop shallots, garlic, thyme, basil, and chard. Set aside. Juice enough lemon for 1 teaspoon and zest enough lemon for ½ teaspoon. Chop mint leaves, chives, and green onions. Seed and dice cucumber. Toss yogurt and salt with cucumber, mint leaves, chives, and green onions. Mix well and set aside. Mix lemon zest, turmeric, pepper, and salt with chard mixture. Fold in turkey and mix well. Form patties and roll edges in hemp hearts. Refrigerate patties for one hour. Fry patties in oil over medium heat, about eight minutes per side. Serve patties over a bed of greens, drizzled with sauce.

Serves: 4	**Prep Time:15 mins.**	**Cooking Time:20 mins.**	
Calories:312	**Protein:35.4g**	**Carbs:7.4g**	**Fat:15.5g**

Mind Diet Dinner Recipes

57.Grilled Salmon with Basil and Tomatoes

Ingredients:

2 tsp salt, divided

2 cloves garlic, minced

1 tbsp olive oil, extra virgin

1 salmon filet (whole), weighing about 1 ½ lbs.

2 tomatoes (medium), sliced thinly

1/3 cup plus ¼ cup basil (fresh), thinly sliced and divided

¼ tsp pepper, freshly ground

Directions:

Preheat the grill to medium setting. On a chopping board, mash together ¾ tsp salt and the minced garlic until you form a paste. Transfer to a bowl and add in oil. Coat a foil with cooking spray. Set the salmon (with the skin's side down) on the foil and spread the garlic mix over it. Sprinkle the salmon with 1/3 cup basil.

Top the salmon with the tomato slices and sprinkle with the ground pepper and the remaining ¼ tsp salt. Place the salmon foil on the grill. Cook for 10 to 12 minutes, or until the fish easily flakes. Transfer the salmon from the foil to the serving plate. Sprinkle with ¼ cup basil on top. Serve and enjoy.

Serves: 4	Prep Time:15 mins.		Cooking Time:15 mins.
Calories:248	Protein:35g	Carbs:3g	Fat:10g

58. Fish Tikka

Ingredients:

4 cloves garlic, crushed or finely grated

2 tbsp. ginger root (fresh), finely grated

2 whole red snapper or sea bream (about 2lb/900g each) or 6 fish steaks like salmon or tuna

2 tbsp. olive oil

6 tbsp. yogurt, plain

2 tsp turmeric

3 tsp cumin seed

2 tsp chili powder, mild

Directions:

Use a sharp knife to slit each side of the whole fish's skin (if you're using a whole fish). Mix the garlic and ginger, and season with salt. Rub the spice mix over the whole fish or the fish filets. Mix the yogurt with the spices, seasoning, and oil. Use the mixture marinate the fish. Chill for an hour or more, until you're ready to cook the fish. Cook the fish on the barbecue rack for 6 to 8 minutes for each side. If you're using steaks, cook for 3 to 4 minutes. If you don't want the fish to stick on the rack, you may cook the fish on foil.

Serves: 6	Prep Time:10 mins.		Cooking Time: 16 mins.
Calories:266	Protein:39g	Carbs:4g	Fat:11g

59. Salmon Stew

Ingredients:

3 peppers (mixed), sliced and deseeded

1 tbsp olive oil

2 tsp paprika, smoked

400g baby potatoes, halved and unpeeled

1 onion (large), sliced thinly

2 tsp thyme, dried

2 cloves garlic, sliced

4 filets salmon

1 can (400g) tomatoes, chopped

1 tbsp parsley (to serve), chopped

Directions:

Heat oil in a pan. Add the onion, potatoes, and peppers. Cook for 5 to 8 minutes or until golden. Stir regularly. Add the garlic, paprika, tomatoes, and thyme. Boil. Reduce the heat and then simmer for 12 minutes. If the sauce becomes thick, add a bit of water. Season the vegetable stew and place the salmon, with the skin side down, on top of the vegetables. Cover the pan and simmer for 8 more minutes until the salmon is cooked. If desired, sprinkle with parsley. Serve immediately.

Serves: 4	Prep Time:10 mins.		Cooking Time:25 mins.
Calories:414	Protein:33g	Carbs:29g	Fat:19g

60. Salmon and Roast Asparagus

Ingredients:

2 tbsp olive oil

400g potatoes (large), halved

8 spears asparagus, halved and trimmed

1 tbsp balsamic vinegar

2 handfuls cherry tomatoes

Handful of basil leaves

2 filets salmon, about 5 oz (140g) each

Directions:

Heat oven to 400°F (200°C). In an ovenproof dish, add the potatoes and 1 tbsp olive oil. Roast for about 20 minutes or until the potatoes start to brown. Add in the asparagus. Bake further for 15 minutes. Add in the vinegar and cherry tomatoes and arrange the salmon among the vegetables. Add the rest of the oil and bake for 10 to 15 minutes more or until the salmon is cooked to your preferred doneness. Sprinkle the basil leaves and serve immediately.

Serves: 2	**Prep Time:20 mins.**	**Cooking Time:1 mins.**
Calories:483	**Protein:33g**	**Carbs:34g**	**Fat:25g**

61. Yogurt Chicken

Ingredients:

8 chicken drumsticks, skinless

1 tsp chili powder

142ml container yogurt, natural

1 tbsp. cumin, ground

2 tsp turmeric, ground

1 tbsp. coriander, ground

Directions:

Score each drumstick several times using a sharp knife. In a bowl, mix together the remaining ingredients. Season to taste. Add the drumsticks, coating each drumstick well with the spice mixture. Cover and marinate for 30 minutes. Shake off excess marinade from the chicken. Barbecue the drumsticks for 20 to 25 minutes, while occasionally turning each drumstick. Serve and enjoy.

Serves: 4	**Prep Time:5 mins.**	**Cooking Time: 20-25 mins.**
Calories:229	**Protein:37g**	**Carbs:6g**	**Fat:7g**

62. Chicken with Sweet Potato, Brussels Sprouts, and Apple Skillet

Ingredients:

1-pound skinless, boneless chicken breasts, sliced into 1/2-inch cubes

4 slices thick-cut bacon, sliced into smaller chunks

1 tablespoon olive oil

1/2 teaspoon black pepper

1 teaspoon salt, divided

3 cups trimmed Brussels sprouts, quartered

1 medium peeled sweet potato, sliced into 1/2-inch cubes

2 peeled Granny Smith apples, cored then cubed into ¾-inch pieces

1 medium-sized onion, sliced

4 2 teaspoons minced garlic cloves

1 teaspoon ground cinnamon

2 teaspoons sliced fresh thyme

1 cup reduced-sodium chicken broth, divided

Directions:

Put olive oil in a cast iron or non-stick large skillet on medium-high heat. Place the chicken into the skillet. Sprinkle with ½ teaspoon salt and some black ground pepper. Cook the chicken until golden brown, which takes about 5 minutes. Place the cooked chicken on a plate lined with paper towels to drain excess oil. In the same skillet, put the chopped bacon pieces. Reduce the heat to medium low.

Cook the bacon until the fat is rendered and the bacon turns brown and crispy. This will take around 8 minutes. Transfer the crisp bacon on some paper towels to drain excess fat. Reserve 1 ½ tablespoons of the bacon fat and discard the rest. Raise the heat setting to medium high. Put sweet potatoes into the skillet. Add the onions, Brussels sprouts and ½ teaspoon salt. Cook until the onions start to turn translucent.

This will take about 10 minutes. Add thyme, cinnamon, garlic and apples into the skillet. Stir and cook quickly for another 30 seconds. Pour ½ cup of broth into the skillet. Allow the liquid to boil until it evaporates. This will take only about 2 minutes. Add the cooked chicken and the rest of the broth. Cook everything until the chicken is heated through. Add the bacon and stir quickly. Spoon into serving plates and serve warm.

Serves: 4	Prep Time:20 mins.		Cooking Time: 25 mins.
Calories:319	Protein:32g	Carbs:26g	Fat:11g

63. Alfredo Spinach Lasagna

Ingredients:

Nonstick cooking spray
1 egg, whisked lightly
1 10-ounce package frozen spinach, thawed, drained then chopped
¼ teaspoon ground black pepper
4 garlic cloves, minced

½ cup fat-free milk
1 15-ounce jar light Alfredo sauce
6 lasagna noodles, whole grain
2 cups sliced fresh mushrooms
2 cups shredded carrots
½ cup nutritional yeast

Directions:

Prepare the oven to 350F. Lightly spray cooking oil at the bottom of a rectangular 2-quart baking dish. Mix spinach, pepper, garlic, spinach and egg in a bowl. Get another bowl and mix together milk and Alfredo sauce. Spread ½ cup of milk-Alfredo sauce mixture into the bottom of the greased baking dish. Place 3 uncooked lasagna noodles on top of the sauce.

Take half of the spinach-egg mixture and pour it over the noodles. Sprinkle half of the mushrooms and half of the carrots over the egg mixture. Place the remaining 3 pieces of lasagna noodles on top of the carrots and mushroom layer. Spread the remaining spinach-egg mixture. Place the rest of the mushrooms and carrots on top. Cover everything with the rest of milk-Alfredo sauce mixture. Top with a layer of nutritional yeast. Spray a piece of foil lightly with cooking spray.

Use this to cover the lasagna, with the greased side down on top of the lasagna. Bake in the preheated oven for 60 to 70 minutes. Remove the cover then bake for another 15 to 20 minutes until the top layer turns a light brown. Remove from the oven and set aside for 20 minutes before slicing. Serve warm.

Serves: 8   Prep Time:20 mins.   Cooking Time: 1 hr. 30 mins.
Calories:262   Protein:16g   Carbs:24g   Fat:12g

64. Cumin Roasted Chicken with Broccoli and Fries

Ingredients:

1 3 - ounce chicken breast

1 teaspoon cumin

3 teaspoons olive oil, divided

2 cups broccoli, sliced in large pieces

1 small potato, sliced into thick slices

Salt and ground pepper, in amounts to your taste

Directions:

Prepare the oven to 375F. Mix 1 teaspoon of oil and cumin. Rub this all over the chicken breast. Place broccoli, potatoes and 2 teaspoon of olive oil in a bowl. Season with pepper and some salt. Toss to mix well. Place chicken on a baking sheet. Add the broccoli and fries. Spread the vegetables into an even layer. Bake everything for 30 minutes. Turn the chicken and stir the vegetables once during the baking period. Check if the chicken internal temperature has reached 165F and all the vegetables are tender. Remove from the oven. Transfer into a serving plate.

Serves: 1	Prep Time:15 mins.		Cooking Time: 30 mins.
Calories:484	Protein:40g	Carbs:46g	Fat:18g

65. Chicken with Salad and Walnut-Lemon Vinaigrette

Ingredients:

3 ounces chicken

Juice from 1 lemon

1 tablespoon olive oil

3 cups baby spinach

1 teaspoon Dijon mustard

2 tablespoons walnuts

1 whole-grain roll

Directions:

Broil or grill the chicken until no longer pink on the inside. Rest for a few minutes before slicing. Pour oil and lemon juice into a blender or small food processor. Add the mustard and walnuts. Pulse until the mixture is smooth and mixed well. Place chicken slices and spinach in a bowl. Pour the dressing and toss to coat all the salad ingredients well. Serve on a plate with 1 whole grain roll.

Serves: 1	Prep Time:20 mins.		Cooking Time: 0 mins.
Calories:517	Protein:31g	Carbs:33g	Fat:32g

66.Salmon & Broccoli Penne

Ingredients:

3 ounces whole-grain dry penne pasta

4 ounces salmon

1 1/2 cups broccoli florets

4 tablespoons water or vegetable low-sodium broth

1 lemon, zested, juiced

1 tablespoon melted coconut oil

1 clove garlic, minced

Directions:

Line a broiler pan with foil. Place the salmon on the pan and broil until flaky, about 8 minutes. You may also grill the salmon if you prefer. Cook the pasta according to the package directions, drain and place in a bowl. Warm the broccoli on a non-stick pan for about 4 minutes. Transfer to the bowl of pasta. Toss to mix. Transfer to a serving plate. Place salmon on top. Place melted coconut oil, lemon juice and zest, broth (or water, if preferred) and garlic in a bowl. Mix well. Drizzle the sauce all over everything and serve immediately.

Serves: 1	Prep Time:20 mins.		Cooking Time: 31 mins.
Calories:547	Protein:36g	Carbs:53g	Fat:21g

67.BBQ Salmon with Sweet Potato

Ingredients:

2 tablespoons barbecue sauce

4 ounces salmon

1 garlic clove, minced

2 teaspoons olive oil

3 cups chopped kale

1 small sweet potato

Dash of cinnamon

2 teaspoons maple syrup

Directions:

Grill the salmon. Brush with barbecue sauce just before it thoroughly cooks. Transfer to a plate once done. Put oil in a skillet on medium-high heat. Add kale and garlic. Sauté until tender, about 6 minutes. Transfer to a plate. Wash the dirt off the sweet potato. Prick all over with a fork or knife. Cover with foil and roast or bake until cooked through. Assemble to serve. Place the sweet potato on a serving plate. Arrange the greens on one side then the salmon on another side of the plate. Drizzle the sweet potato with cinnamon and maple syrup. Serve immediately.

Serves: 1	Prep Time:10 mins.		Cooking Time:20 mins.
Calories:469	Protein:31g	Carbs:47g	Fat:18g

68. Fresh Superfood Summer Rolls with Peanut Dipping Sauce

Ingredients:

Easy peanut dipping sauce:
1/4 cup creamy peanut butter
2 teaspoons soy sauce
1 tablespoon hoisin sauce
1 mashed garlic clove
1-2 tablespoons warm water, add more as needed
1 teaspoon chili garlic sauce or Sriracha sauce

Garnish:
crushed peanuts
crushed red pepper

Summer rolls:
10 pieces rice paper spring roll wrappers

1 large cucumber, julienned
1 peeled large carrot, julienned
1/3 cup chopped purple cabbage
1 small red pepper, julienned
1 avocado, sliced
1-ounce cooked rice vermicelli or rice noodles
handful fresh cilantro
5 large pieces green lettuce leaves such as butter lettuce or romaine), torn in half
20 medium peeled cooked shrimp, halved length-wise
sesame seeds for garnish (optional)

Directions:

Place all ingredients, except water and garnish, and for the dipping sauce, in a deep bowl. Whisk together. Slowly add water to the dipping sauce while whisking. Add water just enough to get the consistency you want. Pour dipping sauce into a serving ramekin. Sprinkle the garnish and set aside for later. Put warm water in a large bowl. Dip the rice paper one by one in the warm water. Soak for about 15 to 20 seconds until they are soft, but not soggy.

The wrapper should be soft but slightly firm, not a soggy mess. Place the soaked rice paper wrapper on a flat surface. Arrange carrot sticks, red pepper, a small amount of cabbage and cucumber on one end of the wrapper. Top with a serving of noodles, cilantro and 1-2 slices of avocado. Place half of a lettuce leaf and 4 shrimp slices. Carefully roll to wrap tightly, folding the ends for a neat wrap. Slice in half and arrange on a serving plate. Sprinkle with sesame seeds. Serve with the dipping sauce on the side.

Serves: 10	Prep Time:30 mins.		Cooking Time: 0 mins.
Calories:400	Protein:30g	Carbs:29g	Fat:19g

69. Spicy Thai Peanut Noodles

Ingredients:

12 oz. spaghetti
1 large cucumber, peeled and seeded, chopped into-2-inch square pieces
1 large red bell pepper, sliced into 2-inch square pieces
1 cup matchstick-sized carrots
1/2 cup chopped cilantro
3/4 cup chopped green onions
1/2 cup roasted lightly salted peanuts, chopped roughly
Sesame seeds, for garnishing

Peanut sauce:
1/4 cup warm water
1/2 cup creamy peanut butter
2 tbsp. honey
3 tbsp. soy sauce
2 tbsp. fresh lime juice
2 tbsp. Sriracha
1 tablespoon minced garlic
1 1/2 tbsp. minced peeled fresh ginger
1 tbsp. sesame oil

Directions:

Cook the pasta according to package directions. Drain and rinse with cold water. Set aside. Put all the ingredients for the sauce in a medium mixing bowl. Whisk well until smooth and blended well. Pour sauce over the pasta. Put cucumber, bell pepper, peanuts, cilantro and green onions into the bowl of pasta. Lightly toss the noodles to mix and coat everything well. Serve with a sprinkle of sesame seeds.

Serves: 4-5	Prep Time:20 mins.	Cooking Time: 7 mins.
Calories:390	Protein:17g	Carbs:58g	Fat:10g

70. Creamy Tagliatelle with Salmon and Spinach

Ingredients:

225 g tagliatelle
1 100-g bag spinach leaves, wash and drain excess water

2 180-g cans boneless and skinless flaked pink salmon
100 g reduced-fat sour cream and chive dip
Black pepper, freshly ground

Directions:

Follow the package directions to cook the pasta. While pasta is cooking, put the spinach inside a colander. When the tagliatelle is done, drain it into the colander with the spinach. The hot pasta water will wilt the leaves. Place both the pasta and the spinach back into the pan. Pour the chive-sour cream dip into the pan. Add the salmon into the pan. Stir to mix the ingredients well. Place the pan over heat set to low. Heat the dish until salmon becomes hot. Spoon into serving plates and serve while still hot. Season with pepper and salt according to preferred flavor.

Serves: 4	Prep Time:20 mins.	Cooking Time: 7 mins.
Calories:398	Protein:15g	Carbs:34g	Fat:10.3g

71.Moroccan Flavored Duck Ragu

Ingredients:

2 lemons

2 teaspoons paprika

2 teaspoons olive oil, divided

1 teaspoon ground coriander

1 teaspoon ground turmeric

1/2 teaspoon freshly ground pepper

1/2 teaspoon ground cumin

1/4 teaspoon ground ginger

1 1/2 pounds boneless Duck chops cut into one inch cubes

14 ounces of chicken broth

1 cup diced butternut squash

1/2 cup chopped onions

1 cup sliced carrots

1 cup rinsed chickpeas

2 tablespoons preserved lemon, rinsed and chopped

1/2 cup tomatoes, diced

1 tablespoon tomato paste

2 teaspoons minced garlic

1/4 teaspoon hot sauce

1 pinch ground allspice

1 pinch ground cinnamon

Directions:

In a medium bowl, combine the lemon juice, paprika, 1/2 teaspoon oil, coriander, turmeric, pepper, cumin and 1/4 teaspoon ginger and thoroughly coat the Duck with this mixture. Refrigerate the marinated meat for a minimum of 30 minutes and a maximum of four hours. Over medium-high heat in a non-stick skillet warm the remaining two teaspoons of oil and add the Duck. Cook two to three minutes.

Add the remaining lemon, allspice, cinnamon, hot sauce, garlic, tomato paste, onions, chick peas, tomatoes, carrots, squash and chicken broth. Bring to a boil, stirring frequently, then reduce heat to a simmer and cook until vegetables are tender, stirring occasionally. Duck should be cooked through in approximately 35 minutes. This recipe makes four servings and there are 330 calories in each serving.

Serves: 6	Prep Time:20 mins.		Cooking Time: 35 mins.
Calories:330	Protein:40.9g	Carbs:28.3g	Fat:22.8g

72. Roast Chicken Salad with Shiitake Mushrooms

Ingredients:

150 g cooked roast chicken

½ cup fresh shiitake mushrooms, sliced

2 cups mixed greens

1-2 tablespoons balsamic vinegar

Pinch black pepper, fresh cracked

Lime juice

Directions:

Heat oil in a pan set over a stove on medium heat setting. Add the mushrooms and cook until golden, about 3 to 4 minutes on each side. Place roast chicken on a chopping board and slice as thinly as you can. Set aside. Arrange mixed greens on a shallow serving plate. Pile the chicken slices at the center of the serving plate. Top with sautéed mushrooms. Drizzle lime juice and balsamic vinegar all over everything. Serve with a sprinkle of freshly cracked black pepper.

Serves: 1   **Prep Time:20 mins.**   **Cooking Time:4 mins.**

Calories:443   **Protein:51.6g**   **Carbs:22g**   **Fat:16.4g**

73. Quick Chicken Tikka Masala

Ingredients:

1/4 teaspoon ground turmeric

1/2 teaspoon salt

4 teaspoons garam masala

1-pound chicken tenders

1/2 cup all-purpose flour

6 cloves garlic, minced

4 teaspoons canola oil, divided

4 teaspoons minced fresh ginger

1 large sweet onion, diced

1/3 cup whipping cream

1 28-ounce can, undrained plum tomatoes

1/2 cup chopped fresh cilantro

Directions:

Stir together salt, turmeric and garam masala in a small dish and throw your flour out in another shallow dish. Coat chicken pieces in 1/2 of the spices then flour. In a large skillet over medium heat, warm two teaspoons of the oil. The chicken should be browned for approximately two minutes on each side and then transferred to a plate. Heat the remaining two teaspoons of oil over low heat. Add ginger, onion, garlic and cook, stirring frequently, about five to seven minutes until the mixture begins to brown. Add the remaining spice mix and cook, stirring, approximately one minute and sprinkle the rest of the flour until coated. Add the tomatoes along with their juice and simmer, while stirring with a wooden spoon to break up the tomatoes. Cook three to five minutes, stirring frequently until the onion is tender and the sauce is thick. Add the chicken, cream, and any accumulated juices and stir them over medium-low heat until simmering. Chicken should be cooked through in approximately five minutes. Garnish with cilantro.

Serves: 4   **Prep Time:20 mins.**   **Cooking Time:21 mins.**

Calories:310   **Protein:17.7g**   **Carbs:44.6g**   **Fat:6.9g**

74. Chicken Stir Fry

Ingredients:

1-pound chicken tenders, sliced

1 red bell pepper, sliced

1 green bell pepper, sliced

3 tablespoons olive oil

1 cup mushrooms, sliced

1 red onion, sliced

2 teaspoons ground cumin

2 teaspoons ground turmeric

1 teaspoon garlic powder

Directions:

Heat the olive oil in a wok or a large skillet. Add the chicken and cook until it begins to brown on each side and is hot throughout. Remove the chicken, leaving the juices in the pan and add the vegetables. When the vegetables are nearly done cooking, put the chicken back in the wok and combine. Add the cumin, turmeric and garlic powder. Toss everything together until combined and hot. Serve over rice or noodles.

Serves: 4   **Prep Time:20 mins.**   **Cooking Time:21 mins.**

Calories:385   **Protein:24g**   **Carbs:13.6g**   **Fat:4.4g**

75. Grilled Salmon

Ingredients:

4 wild-caught salmon filets, 6 ounces each

8 cherry tomatoes, cut in half

1/2 red onion, sliced into rings

1 garlic clove

1/2 teaspoon red pepper flakes

1 teaspoon white wine vinegar

2 tablespoons olive oil

1 tablespoon ground turmeric

Directions:

In a large bowl or a shallow baking dish, whisk together the oil, vinegar, garlic and turmeric. Place the salmon in the dish and marinate the fish for at least 30 minutes in the refrigerator. Flip the fillets over at least once so both sides can get coated with the oil and the spices. Heat your grill. Cook the salmon on the grill for 8-10 minutes, until cooked through. Top with chopped tomatoes and onions to serve. This recipe makes four servings and there are 372 calories in each serving.

Serves: 4   **Prep Time:15 mins.**   **Cooking Time:10 mins.**

Calories:372   **Protein:4.8g**   **Carbs:24.5g**   **Fat:7.2g**

76. Chicken Stir-Fry

Ingredients

2 cups cooked quinoa

Ginger (1/2-inch, peeled, sliced thinly)

2 cloves garlic, peeled, sliced thinly

1 bunch radishes, quartered

1/2 cup yellow onion, finely chopped

1/2-pound sirloin, thinly sliced

1/2 tsp curry powder

1/8 tsp Himalayan salt

1/8 tsp black pepper

1/2 tsp turmeric

2 Tbs coconut oil

1 Tbs honey

2 Tbs tamari

1 Tbs balsamic vinegar

1 cup snow peas

1/4 tsp salt

Directions

In a medium bowl, combine your spices. Add sirloin and mix well until evenly coated.

Heat 1 tablespoon coconut oil in a large skillet over medium-high heat. Add sirloin in an even layer, and cook undisturbed until browned on bottom, about one minute. Flip and cook for an additional thirty seconds. Remove from skillet and set aside. Add 1 tablespoon of coconut oil to the skillet, reduce to low heat, and cook radishes, onion, garlic and ginger then stir frequently, until onion becomes translucent (about 6 minutes).

Add honey and return to medium heat; cook for about 2 minutes or until radishes are fully glazed. Add balsamic vinegar and tamari then simmer until thickened (about 2 minutes). Add snow peas and radish greens then season well. Continue cooking, while stirring, until greens begin to wilt. Add chicken and stir until warm. Serve over quinoa.

Serves: 4	Prep Time:15 mins.		Cooking Time:15 mins.
Calories:493	Protein:25.3g	Carbs:65.4g	Fat:14.8g

77. Seafood Curry

Ingredients

2 large shallots, thinly sliced
1 clove garlic, minced
1 Tbs ginger, minced
1/2 lime, juiced
2 medium carrots
1 cup cilantro. chopped
1-pound shrimp (peeled, deveined)
Quinoa (6 servings, cooked)
2 Tbs coconut oil
1/2-pound scallops

2 Tbs curry powder
1 tsp turmeric
2 stems lemon grass
1 Tbs maple syrup (optional)
1 can coconut milk
1/2 tsp Himalayan salt
1/4 tsp pepper
1/4 cup basil leaves
1/2-pound snow peas

Directions

In a saucepan over medium heat, sauté shallots in coconut oil until soft. Add garlic, shrimp, scallops, curry powder, turmeric, and ginger, and cook for another few minutes, stirring frequently. Add lemon grass and carrots, and cook for a few minutes more, turning shrimp and scallops. Add maple syrup, coconut milk, salt, pepper, and lime juice, and bring to a simmer, cooking a further ten minutes. Stir in snow peas and basil. Spoon curry over quinoa; garnish with cilantro.

Serves: 4   Prep Time:20 mins.   Cooking Time:16 mins.
Calories:272   Protein:32.6g   Carbs:17.9g   Fat:8.5g

78.Golden Baked Chicken

Ingredients

1-inch piece fresh ginger, grated
1/3 cup balsamic vinegar
1/3 cup blackstrap molasses
1/4 tsp pepper
1½ tsp red miso
1 tsp rice wine
1/2 tsp turmeric

1 Tbs water
2 pounds boneless, skinless chicken breasts
1 bunch green onions, chopped
1/3 cup cilantro, chopped
Quinoa (4 servings) cooked
2 cups mixed greens

Directions

In a small pot on medium heat, add pepper, ginger, molasses and vinegar then allow to boil; lower the heat then simmer for 10 minutes. Combine water, turmeric, rice wine and miso then stir into the molasses mixture. Set to cool. Separate your marinade in two and set half aside. Pour the other half over your chicken and set to marinate for at least 2 hours. Remove chicken from marinade and discard the used marinade. Preheat oven to 350 degrees. Bake chicken, covered, in an oiled baking dish for 45 minutes or until fully cooked. Serve with your quinoa and greens. Top with unused marinade, cilantro and green onions.

Serves: 4   **Prep Time:20 mins.**   **Cooking Time:45 mins.**
Calories:505   **Protein:21.9g**   **Carbs:73.7g**   **Fat:13.1g**

79. Mini-Meatloaf

Ingredients

1 zucchini

2 carrots

1/3 cup onion

1 leaf kale

3 cloves garlic

2 Tbs fresh thyme or 2 tsp dried

2 Tbs coconut oil

1½ lbs. ground turkey

1 large egg

1/2 cup almond flour

1 tsp Himalayan salt

1 tsp cumin

1 tsp turmeric

1/4 tsp allspice

1/4 tsp black pepper

3/4 cup tomato sauce

1 Tbs coconut sugar

1 Tbs blackstrap molasses

2 tsp apple cider vinegar

1/2 tsp onion powder

1/4 tsp Himalayan salt

Directions

Grate zucchini and carrots. Finely chop onion and kale. Press or mince garlic. Chop thyme, if using fresh. Preheat oven to 350 degrees. Prepare muffin tins with liners or oil. Heat coconut oil in a large skillet; sauté onion, zucchini, and carrot until tender. Add garlic and sauté a few minutes longer; allow to cool slightly. Combine sautéed ingredients in a large bowl, stir in other ingredients, and mix well. Divide mixture among eight muffin tins, press. Bake for forty-five minutes. Combine ingredients; pour over each mini-meatloaf. Bake an additional fifteen minutes. Serve mini-meatloaves with additional sauce, if desired.

Serves: 4   **Prep Time:20 mins.**   **Cooking Time:1 hr.**

Calories:428   **Protein:36.3g**   **Carbs:21.9g**   **Fat:21.5g**

80. Roasted Turkey Tenderloin and Vegetables

Ingredients

3 pounds turkey tenderloin
1 cup balsamic vinegar
1½ cup extra virgin olive oil
3 Tbs Dijon mustard
1 Tbs honey
2 cloves garlic
1 head cauliflower

2 sweet potatoes
3 Tbs extra virgin olive oil
1/2 tsp Himalayan salt
1 tsp turmeric
4 Tbs fresh basil
1/2 tsp salt
1/4 tsp pepper

Directions

Whisk vinegar, oil, mustard, and honey. Marinate turkey in this mixture for 2 hours. Peel and mince garlic. Chop cauliflower into bite-sized pieces. Thinly slice sweet potatoes. Preheat oven to 350 degrees. In a medium bowl, mix oil, salt, turmeric, and garlic. Place cauliflower on a rimmed cookie sheet, drizzle oil mixture over the florets, toss to coat evenly. Roast, stirring occasionally, thirty-five to forty-five minutes, until golden brown and tender. Put turkey and sweet potatoes in a baking dish; sprinkle with basil, salt, and pepper. Cover and bake fifteen to twenty minutes or until tender. Slice turkey and serve with cauliflower and sweet potatoes

Serves: 8   **Prep Time:20 mins.**   **Cooking Time:1 hr.**
Calories:1042   **Protein:98.9g**   **Carbs:20.5g**   **Fat:59.4g**

81. Moroccan Chicken

Ingredients

Sprouted rice
1 onion
2 cloves garlic
1/2 cup dates
2 carrot
2 large zucchinis
1/4 cup fresh parsley
1 inch ginger
4 cups chickpeas, soaked overnight (or 2 cans)
2 pounds boneless, skinless chicken breast

2 Tbs coconut oil
2 tsp thyme leaves
1 tsp turmeric
1/2 tsp cinnamon
1/2 tsp pepper
1/2 tsp salt
1 tsp ground coriander
2 bay leaves
1½ quarts chicken stock
1 cup plain Greek yogurt.

Directions

Cook rice according to package directions to make four servings; refrigerate until serving time. Roughly chop onion, garlic, dates, carrot, zucchini, and parsley. Grate ginger. Rinse and drain chickpeas. Cube chicken. Brown chicken in coconut oil over medium heat. Remove from pan, and place in slow cooker. Sauté onion, garlic, and 2 tablespoons chicken stock until onion is translucent, scraping browned bits. Add to slow cooker. Add remaining ingredients (except zucchini and rice) to slow cooker and cook on low for eight hours or high four hours. Add zucchini in at the last hour. Warm rice. Remove bay leaves; serve over rice with a dollop of yogurt.

Serves: 4   Prep Time:25 mins.   Cooking Time:8 hrs.
Calories:825   Protein:32.5g   Carbs:93g   Fat:37.6g

82.Smothered Chicken and Sweet Potatoes

Ingredients

Quinoa, cooked, 6 servings

2 pounds boneless skinless chicken, sliced

1-pound cremini mushrooms, sliced

1 shallot, sliced

1 sweet potato, diced

2 Tbs coconut oil

1 cup chicken broth

1 cup coconut milk

1 cup chicken broth

1 tsp Himalayan salt

1 tsp black pepper

1 Tbs capers

2 cups baby spinach

Directions

Preheat oven to 350 degrees. In a skillet, add oil and brown chicken on all sides. Add shallot, mushrooms and then continue to cook a bit longer, while stirring. In a small bowl, whisk in a cup of broth and coconut milk. Add sweet potato and chicken mix to a baking dish, and season to taste. Pour in broth and coconut milk on top. Cover and bake twenty minutes, or until sweet potatoes are soft. Add baby spinach into the chicken mixture. Serve over quinoa, and top with capers.

Serves: 6   **Prep Time:25 mins.**   **Cooking Time:30 mins.**

Calories:392   **Protein:55.3g**   **Carbs:5.8g**   **Fat:15.7g**

MIND Diet Vegetarian & Side Dish Recipes

83.Black Bean and Sweet Potato Chili
Ingredients:

1 sweet potato (medium-large), peeled and diced

1 tbsp. plus 2 tbsp. olive oil, extra virgin

1 onion (large), diced

2 tbsp chili powder

4 garlic cloves, minced

4 tsp cumin, ground

½ tsp chipotle chili, ground

2 ½ cups water

¼ tsp salt

1 can (14 oz) tomatoes, diced

2 cans (15 oz) black beans, rinsed

½ cup cilantro (fresh), chopped

4 tsp lime juice

Directions:

In a Dutch oven on medium-high, heat the oil. Add the onion and sweet potato. Cook for about 4 minutes, stirring often, or until the onion is starting to soften. Add the chili powder, garlic, chipotle, salt, and cumin. Cook for 30 seconds, constantly stirring. Add water, cover, and simmer for 10 to 12 minutes or until the sweet potato becomes tender. Add the lime juice, tomatoes, and beans. Turn up the heat and simmer. Stir often. Reduce the heat and simmer for 5 minutes, or until the sauce is slightly reduced. Add the cilantro. Ladle into bowls. Serve and enjoy.

Serves: 4	Prep Time:25 mins.		Cooking Time:15 mins.
Calories:323	Protein:13g	Carbs:55g	Fat:8g

84.Broccoli with Herbs
Ingredients:

1 mint bunch (small), leaves chopped

300g regular broccoli or Tender stem broccoli

2 tbsp pine nuts, toasted

1 jar (145g) basil pesto

Directions:

Steam the broccoli until tender or for 5 to 8 minutes. Meanwhile, add the mint to the pesto. Stir to combine. Place the broccoli on a serving dish. Drizzle the broccoli with the pesto. Sprinkle the pine nuts on top. Serve and enjoy.

Serves: 4	Prep Time:5 mins.		Cooking Time: 8 mins.
Calories:178	Protein:11g	Carbs:3g	Fat:14g

85. Chickpeas with Spinach & Tomatoes

Ingredients:

1 onion (red), sliced

1 tbsp vegetable oil

2 cloves garlic, chopped

2 red chilies (mild), sliced thinly

½ fresh ginger root (finger-length), shredded

½ tsp turmeric

1 tsp cumin, ground

¾ tsp garam masala

2 tsp tomato puree

4 tomatoes, chopped

200g baby spinach leaves

1 can (400g) chickpeas, drained and rinsed

Naan bread or rice, to serve

Directions:

In a wok on low heat, heat the oil and fry onion until it becomes soft. Add the ginger, chilies, and garlic and for 5 minutes more until the garlic is toasted lightly and the onions are golden. Add the garam masala, cumin, and turmeric. Over low heat, stir for a few seconds. Add the tomatoes and the tomato puree. Simmer for about 5 minutes. Add the chickpeas together with 300ml of water, and simmer for about 10 minutes. Add in the spinach leaves and wilt them. Season and serve with naan or rice.

Serves: 4	Prep Time:10 mins.		Cooking Time: 25 mins.
Calories:145	Protein:7g	Carbs:17g	Fat:6g

86. Sage and Broccoli Pasta

Ingredients:

140g spaghetti, quick-cook

3 tbsp olive oil

140g regular broccoli or Tender stem broccoli, trimmed and cut to 2" lengths

2 shallots, sliced

¼ tsp chilies, crushed

1 clove garlic, chopped finely

12 leaves sage, shredded

Directions:

Boil quick-cook spaghetti for one minute. Put in the broccoli and cook further for 4 minutes. Meanwhile, heat the oil and add the garlic and shallots. Cook gently for 5 minutes or until golden. Add the sage and chilies and cook gently further for 2 minutes. Drain the spaghetti. Add it into the shallot mixture. Serve hot and enjoy.

Serves: 2	Prep Time:5 mins.		Cooking Time: 12 mins.
Calories:419	Protein:12g	Carbs:55g	Fat:19g

87.Roasted Cauliflower with Turmeric and Lemon Pepper

Ingredients:

1 whole cauliflower

1 teaspoon salt

1/4 cup olive oil

1 teaspoon lemon pepper

2 teaspoons ground turmeric

2 teaspoons curry powder

Directions:

Preheat oven to 450 degrees and use heavy duty foil to line a large baking sheet. Cut cauliflower into ¾ inch steaks. Mix spices, salt and oil in a generous size zip-lock bag. Coat cauliflower pieces with mixture. Place on baking sheet and roast for approximately 20 minutes.

Serves: 4   **Prep Time:5 mins.**   **Cooking Time:20 mins.**

Calories:162   **Protein:0.5g**   **Carbs:2.6g**   **Fat:13.7g**

88.Roasted Chili Potatoes

Ingredients:

1-pound potatoes, cleaned and chopped

1/2 cup olive oil

2 garlic cloves, chopped

1 yellow onion, chopped

2 stalks celery, chopped

1 teaspoon cumin seeds

1 teaspoon turmeric

1 teaspoon ground coriander

2 teaspoons ground chili powder

Directions:

Heat an oven to 400 degrees. Pour the potatoes, celery, onion and garlic into a large roasting pan or baking dish. Pour the olive oil over the potatoes and vegetables, stirring to make sure everything is coated. Add the cumin, turmeric, coriander and chili powder. Toss together until combined. Heat in the oven for 40-50 minutes, until potatoes are cooked and beginning to get crispy.

Serves: 4   **Prep Time:5 mins.**   **Cooking Time:50 mins.**

Calories:325   **Protein:3g**   **Carbs:23.7g**   **Fat:29.8 g**

89. Turmeric Latkes with Applesauce

Ingredients:

1/2 teaspoon ground turmeric

1 tablespoon canola oil

2 teaspoons grated fresh ginger

1 cup unsweetened applesauce

1/2 teaspoon ground cloves

2 cups peeled, shredded potatoes

1 teaspoon ground cumin

1-2 green chilies, chopped fine and steamed

1 small finely chopped onion

3 tablespoons finely chopped cilantro

1/2 cup chickpea flour

1 teaspoon kosher or sea salt

2 large eggs, slightly beaten

2 tablespoons canola oil, divided

Directions:

Prepare sauce by heating one tablespoon oil over medium heat in a small skillet. Add ginger and cook, stirring, 30 to 60 seconds. Stir in cloves and turmeric and cook approximately one more minute. Place the applesauce in a small bowl and stir in the spices. Preheat oven to 200 degrees. Prepare Latkes – In a large bowl, thoroughly mix chilis, onion, potatoes, cilantro, salt, flour, cumin, eggs and turmeric. Heat one tablespoon oil in a large griddle over medium heat. Take a generous tablespoon of the mixture and place on the griddle and flatten into a three-inch disk. Make as many latkes as possible without overcrowding the pan. Cook until bottoms are crispy and tops golden brown, usually three to five minutes. Briefly drain on a plate lined with paper towels and transfer to the preheated oven to keep warm. Serve with seasoned applesauce.

Serves: 6	Prep Time:5 mins.		Cooking Time:50 mins.
Calories:185	Protein:3.9g	Carbs:19.5g	Fat:9.2 g

90. Spicy Smashed Cauliflower

Ingredients:

1 whole cauliflower

4 tablespoons olive oil

2 teaspoons chili powder

2 teaspoons ground turmeric

2 teaspoons ground cumin

2 teaspoons ground coriander

1 teaspoon black pepper

1 teaspoon white pepper

Salt to taste

Directions:

Boil a large pot of water on the stove and add a little salt to the water. Cook the head of cauliflower until it softens. In a frying pan, add olive oil and stir the spices into the mixture until combined. Drain the cauliflower and return to pot. Pour the oil and spices over the cauliflower and mash with a hand masher. Salt to taste before you serve.

Serves: 4	Prep Time:5 mins.		Cooking Time:13 mins.
Calories:145	Protein:0.7g	Carbs:3g	Fat:14 g

91. Tandoori Tofu

Ingredients:

1 teaspoon salt, divided
2 teaspoons paprika
1/2 teaspoon ground coriander
1/2 teaspoon ground cumin
3 tablespoons extra-virgin olive oil
1/4 teaspoon ground turmeric

2/3 cup nonfat plain yogurt
1 tablespoon lime juice
1 tablespoon minced garlic
2 14-ounce packages tofu, drained
6 tablespoons chopped fresh cilantro or sliced scallions for garnish

Directions:

Preheat grill to high. Combine paprika, turmeric, cumin, coriander, 1/2 teaspoon salt in a bowl and over medium heat, warm oil in a small skillet. Add spice mixture, lime juice and garlic and cook, stirring frequently about one minute until fragrant and sizzling, then immediately remove from burner. Slice each block of tofu crosswise into six pieces and drain excess water.

Brush the tofu slices with three tablespoons of the spiced oil and sprinkle them with the remaining 1/2 teaspoon of salt. Grill the tofu for two or three minutes on each side. In a small bowl combine the remaining spiced oil and yogurt. Serve the tofu with the yogurt sauce and if desired, garnish with cilantro or scallions.

Serves: 6	Prep Time:20 mins.		Cooking Time:13 mins.
Calories:175	Protein:24.1g	Carbs:16.9g	Fat:30.8 g

92. Turmeric Rice

Ingredients:

2 tablespoons coconut oil
1 minced garlic clove
1 drop thyme
1/2 chopped onion
1 bay leaf

1 cup basmati rice
1 1/2 cups chicken broth
1 tablespoon turmeric
Salt and pepper to taste

Directions:

Melt 1 tablespoon coconut oil in a large saucepan, add garlic and onion and cook until tender. Add turmeric and rice and stir to coat. Add remaining ingredients and allow mixture to come to a rolling boil, cover and simmer 15 minutes. Stir in remaining coconut oil and discard bay leaf.

Serves: 4	Prep Time:10 mins.		Cooking Time:25 mins.
Calories:255	Protein:24g	Carbs:19.5g	Fat:19.3g

93. Rice with Broccoli and Kale

Ingredients:

1 cup basmati rice

1 1/2 cups chicken broth

2 tablespoons olive oil

1 cup chopped kale

1 cup chopped broccoli

1 clove garlic, minced

1 tablespoon turmeric

1 teaspoon dried thyme

Salt and pepper

Directions:

Add oil to a saucepan then stir in the kale and broccoli until the vegetables are soft and cooked. Add the basmati rice, thyme and turmeric, then stir until everything is coated. Add the chicken broth to the saucepan and bring the entire mixture to a boil, stirring to prevent sticking. Cover and simmer for 15 minutes. Let the pot sit for five minutes after you remove it from heat, and then serve. Add salt and pepper to taste.

Serves: 4	Prep Time:10 mins.	Cooking Time:25 mins.
Calories:280	Protein:24.3g	Carbs:18.9g	Fat:19.3g

94. Red Lentil, Turmeric and Cumin Mash

Ingredients:

1 chopped medium onion

1 tablespoon olive oil

1 chopped garlic clove

2 teaspoons turmeric

1 bay leaf

2 teaspoons curry powder

1/2 teaspoon cumin seed

2 teaspoons black mustard seeds

1 tablespoon of chopped black pepper

1/2 teaspoon chili paste

8 cups red lentils, rinsed and drained

1 tablespoon of fresh chopped coriander

1 1/2 cups vegetable stock

Directions:

Heat oil in a saucepan over medium heat and add the bay leaf, garlic and onion. Turn heat to low and cook for five minutes. Add cumin, mustard seeds, turmeric, chili paste and curry powder and cook for an additional minute. Add stock and lentils. Bring to boil and allow to simmer for 15-20 minutes until stock is absorbed and lentils tender. Mash coarsely and serve.

Serves: 6	Prep Time:10 mins.	Cooking Time:26 mins.
Calories:250	Protein:63.8g	Carbs:16.9g	Fat:59.3g

95. Butternut Squash Curry

Ingredients

1 cup finely chopped shallot

2 cloves thinly sliced garlic

2-pound butternut squash, peeled, cleaned and diced

1 can chickpeas, drained and rinsed

1/2 cup cilantro, chopped

2 cups cooked quinoa

1 Tbs coconut oil

1 can coconut milk

3 Tbs mild curry paste, or more to taste

1 tsp salt

1 lime, sliced into wedges

Directions

In a large enough pot on medium heat, melt coconut oil. Add shallot and garlic, and cook, stirring frequently, until shallot is soft, about three minutes. Add salt, curry paste and coconut milk then allow to boil. Add squash; return to boil. Reduce heat and simmer, uncovered, fifteen minutes or until squash is tender. Stir in chickpeas and cilantro then cook while stirring until warmed all the way through. Serve curry with a squeeze of lime over a bed of quinoa.

Serves: 4   Prep Time:15 mins.   Cooking Time:18 mins.

Calories:493   Protein:25.3g   Carbs:65.4g   Fat:14.8g

96. Cauliflower Hash

Ingredients

1 cauliflower

1 bunch green onions

1 small zucchini

3 cloves garlic

1-inch ginger

1/4 cup cilantro

1 lime

2 Tbs coconut oil

1-pound ground turkey

1 tsp turmeric

1 tsp ground cumin

1/4 tsp black pepper

1/2 tsp Himalayan salt

Directions

Core and grate the cauliflower, dice the onions and zucchini, peel and mince or chop the garlic, and grate the ginger. Chop the cilantro and slice the lime into wedges. Heat 1 tablespoon coconut oil in a large skillet over medium heat. Add cauliflower, garlic, and onion. Cook, stirring occasionally, for eight to ten minutes. Remove from pan and set aside. Heat remaining oil, and cook turkey along with the turmeric, cumin, pepper, salt, and ginger for five minutes. Add zucchini and cook a further three to five minutes. Toss turkey mixture with cauliflower and cilantro and serve with a squeeze of lime.

Serves: 4   Prep Time:15 mins.   Cooking Time:20 mins.

Calories:617   Protein:22.1g   Carbs:2.6g   Fat:57.4g

97.Curried Quinoa and Veggies

Ingredients

1 cup quinoa	1 tsp turmeric
1-inch piece ginger	2½ cups vegetable stock
1 Tbs coconut oil	1 can coconut milk
1 chopped shallot	1/2 tsp salt
2 diced carrots	1/4 tsp pepper
1 Tbs green curry paste	1 handful fresh peas

Directions

Rinse quinoa, soak for fifteen minutes in cold water, and drain. Grate the ginger. Curry
Heat coconut oil in a large saucepan over medium heat. Sauté until the shallot is translucent. Add ginger and carrots; sauté a few minutes more. Add curry paste, turmeric, and a splash of stock. Increase heat, bring to a boil, then reduce heat and simmer for five minutes. Add quinoa, coconut milk, and vegetable stock. Increase heat, bring to a boil, then reduce heat, cover, and simmer for a further twenty minutes, or until quinoa is done. Season with salt and pepper as desired, garnish with peas, and serve warm or at room temperature.

Serves: 4 **Prep Time:45 mins.** **Cooking Time:8 mins.**
Calories:217 **Protein:21.6g** **Carbs:13.4g** **Fat:10.1g**

98. Curried Vegetable Sauté

Ingredients

Couscous

2 Tbs cashews

1 yellow onion

2 cups savoy cabbage

1/4 cup cilantro

1 sweet potato

4 dates

1 Tbs fresh ginger

3 cloves garlic

1 lime

1 can chickpeas

1 Tbs coconut oil

1½ tsp cumin

1 Tbs coriander

1 tsp turmeric

1/4 tsp black pepper

2 cups vegetable broth

1 can coconut milk

Directions

Cook couscous according to package directions to make four servings. Chop cashews, and toast them in a dry skillet over medium heat, stirring frequently. Set aside. Chop onion, cabbage, and cilantro. Finely dice the sweet potato. Pit and chop dates. Grate ginger. Mince or press garlic. Cut lime into wedges. Rinse and drain chickpeas. Sauté onion, cumin, coriander, turmeric, and pepper in a large skillet over medium heat until onion begins to soften. Stir in cabbage, sweet potato, chickpeas, dates, ginger, and garlic. Sauté an additional five minutes. Add broth, reduce heat, and cover. Simmer until sweet potatoes are tender, about ten minutes, stirring occasionally. Stir in coconut milk, warm a few minutes longer. Serve over couscous topped with cashews, cilantro, and a squeeze of lime.

Serves: 4	Prep Time:15 mins.		Cooking Time:28 mins.
Calories:82	Protein:1.7g	Carbs:12.3g	Fat:3.8g

99. Harvest Kuri Curry

Ingredients

1/2 cup shredded coconut
1 medium red kuri squash
1 Tbs coconut oil
1 sweet onion
2 cloves garlic
2 inches fresh ginger
3 cups cauliflower
2 cups kale
1 lime
Quinoa
2 Tbs coconut oil

2 tsp ground coriander
1/2 tsp salt
1 tsp turmeric
1 tsp ground mustard
1 tsp chili powder
1/2 tsp cayenne, or to taste
1/2 tsp cumin
1/4 tsp cardamom
2 cups vegetable stock
1 can coconut milk

Directions

Preheat oven to 350 degrees. Toast coconut in a dry skillet over medium heat for two to three minutes, stirring constantly. Cut squash in half; spread 1 tablespoon coconut oil on cut sides. Place in a baking dish cut sides down, and bake for thirty to forty-five minutes, or until tender. While squash is baking, prep other ingredients. Peel and dice onion. Peel and press or mince garlic. Grate ginger. Chop cauliflower and kale.

Juice lime. Following package instructions, make enough quinoa for four servings. Sauté onion, garlic, and ginger in 2 tablespoons coconut oil in a dutch oven or soup pot over medium heat. When onion is translucent, add cauliflower, spices, and vegetable stock. Simmer twenty minutes, or until cauliflower is al dente. When squash is cooked, scoop out flesh and add to cauliflower. Stir in kale, coconut milk, and lime juice. Simmer until kale is bright green and tender, stirring occasionally. Ladle over quinoa, and sprinkle toasted coconut on top.

Serves: 4   **Prep Time:30 mins.**   **Cooking Time: 45 mins.**
Calories:314.7   **Protein:10.1g**   **Carbs:41.7g**   **Fat:13.8g**

100. Sweet Potato and Brussels Sprout Hash

Ingredients

3 eggs

2 sprigs rosemary

1 bunch green onions

1/2-pound brussels sprouts

2 portabella mushrooms

2 cloves garlic

2 inches fresh ginger

1 sweet potato

1 lemon

5 Tbs coconut oil

1 Tbs turmeric

4 eggs

2 Tbs coconut oil

2 tsp pepper

1/2 tsp salt

Directions

Separate eggs; set aside. Stem rosemary, and chop. Chop green onions, brussels sprouts, and mushrooms. Mince or press garlic. Press ginger. Peel and dice sweet potato. Juice lemon. Melt coconut oil in a small saucepan over medium heat. Add rosemary and turmeric; cook for a minute or two. Remove from heat and set aside.

To prepare the sauce, combine egg yolks with 1/4 cup of water and lemon juice in the top part of a double boiler or a small bowl that will fit over the saucepan of simmering water. Whisk mixture for several minutes, until it begins to thicken. Slowly add coconut oil mixture and continue to whisk until well mixed and sauce is thickened. Remove from heat and set aside. Sauté onions, garlic, and ginger in a skillet over medium heat.

While onions are cooking, heat 2 inches of water in a small saucepan or double boiler until simmering. When onions are soft, add sweet potatoes and 1/4 cup water. Cover and cook a further eight to ten minutes, stirring frequently. When sweet potatoes are soft, add brussels sprouts and portabellas and cook four to five minutes longer, stirring frequently. Season with salt and pepper. Prepare eggs as desired; if scrambling, mix in separated whites to avoid waste. Divide hash among plates; serve each with an egg and sauce.

Serves: 6	Prep Time:15 mins.		Cooking Time: 30 mins.
Calories:177.7	Protein:4.5g	Carbs:26.4g	Fat:7.1g

101. *Harvest Casserole*

Ingredients

3 cups chicken stock
1 cup amaranth
1 medium winter squash
1/2 cup dates
2 Tbs almond flour
1 tsp salt
1 tsp freshly ground pepper
1 tsp cinnamon
1/2 tsp ground ginger

1/2 tsp nutmeg
1 tsp turmeric
1 Tbs fresh thyme leaves or 1 tsp dried
2 Tbs maple syrup
1 cup chicken stock
1/2 cup coconut cream
1/4 cup pumpkin seeds
1 Tbs coconut flakes

Directions

In a large saucepan, bring chicken stock to a boil. Add the amaranth, reduce heat, and simmer forty minutes or until the liquid is absorbed. Preheat oven to 350 degrees. Grease a 9 x 12 baking dish or two-quart casserole. Peel, seed, and dice the winter squash. Chop dates; toss with almond flour to coat. Place squash and date in baking dish. Combine dry herbs and spices, and sprinkle on top along with fresh thyme, if using. Combine maple syrup, 1 cup chicken stock, and coconut cream, then pour over ingredients in baking dish. Bake covered for forty-five minutes. Uncover, sprinkle with pumpkin seeds and coconut flakes, increase heat to 400 degrees, and bake an additional ten minutes. Spoon casserole over a bed of amaranth.

Serves: 4   Prep Time:20 mins.   Cooking Time: 1 hr.
Calories:367.7   Protein:20g   Carbs:36.6g   Fat:15.1g

102. Stuffed Acorn Squash

Ingredients

1/3 cup toasted pumpkin seeds

1 finely chopped shallot

3 cups cooked black beans or 2 15-oz. cans, drained and rinsed

2 Tbs chopped cilantro

Quinoa

4 acorn squash

3 Tbs extra virgin olive oil

1 Tbs ground cumin

1 tsp ground oregano

1/2 tsp salt

1/4 cup water or vegetable or chicken stock

2 cups chopped fresh spinach

Directions

Preheat oven to 375 degrees. Toast pumpkin seeds in a dry skillet over medium heat. Peel and finely chop shallot. Drain and rinse black beans. Chop cilantro. Cook, according to package directions, enough quinoa to make 1½ cups cooked grains. Lightly coat large baking sheet with oil or cooking spray. Cut squash in half tip-to-stem. Scoop out and discard seeds. Place squash cut side down on baking sheet. Bake until tender, about forty-five minutes. Heat olive oil in medium saucepan over medium heat. Add shallot and seasonings. Sauté, stirring often, until shallot softens, about five minutes.

Stir in water, beans, quinoa, and spinach. Simmer about ten minutes, mashing and stirring mixture with back of a fork. If beans seem too dry, add small amounts of water until desired consistency is reached. Adjust seasonings. Remove pan from heat. With back of the fork, continue to break up bean mixture to desired consistency. When the squash is tender, remove and reduce oven temperature to 325 degrees. Fill squash halves with bean mixture. Garnish squash with cilantro and pumpkin seeds.

Serves: 4	Prep Time:15 mins.		Cooking Time: 45 mins.
Calories:153.7	Protein:5.6g	Carbs:26.3g	Fat:4.3g

Mind Diet Soups, Stews & Salad Recipes

103. *Avocado and Chicken Salad with Balsamic Dressing*
Ingredients:

85g blueberries
1 clove garlic
2 tsp balsamic vinegar
1 tbsp rapeseed oil, extra virgin
1 avocado (deseeded), sliced and peeled

1 beetroot (large), cooked and chopped finely
1 bag (85g) baby leaf salad, mixed
125g frozen or fresh baby broad beans
175g chicken, cooked

Directions:

Chop the garlic finely. In a large salad bowl, mash half of the blueberries with the vinegar, oil, and a dash of black pepper. Boil the beans until tender or for about 5 minutes. Drain, but do not skin the beans. Add the garlic to the blueberry dressing. Stir. Add the beans and the rest of the blueberries with the avocado, beetroot, chicken, and salad. Toss lightly. To serve, place the salad on shallow bowls or plates. Serve and enjoy.

Serves: 2	Prep Time:15 mins.	Cooking Time: 5 mins.
Calories:402	Protein:34g	Carbs:18g	Fat:19g

104. *Avocado, Mango, and Raspberry Salad*
Ingredients:

¼ cup olive oil, extra virgin
1 ½ cups raspberries (fresh), divided
1 garlic clove (small), chopped coarsely
¼ cup red wine vinegar
¼ tsp kosher salt
1/8 tsp pepper, freshly ground

8 cups salad greens, mixed
1 ripe avocado (small), diced
1 mango (ripe), diced
½ cup red onion, sliced thinly
¼ cup toasted hazelnuts (chopped) or almonds (sliced)

Directions:

In a blender, puree ½ cup raspberries, vinegar, oil, salt, garlic, and pepper. Process until combined well. In a large bowl, combine the mango, greens, onion, and avocado. Add the dressing and toss gently. Distribute the salad among 5 plates. Sprinkle with nuts and top with the rest of the raspberries.

Serves: 5	Prep Time:25 mins.	Cooking Time: 0 mins.
Calories:229	Protein:3g	Carbs:21g	Fat:16g

105. Squash, Barley, and Orange Salad

Ingredients:

1 kg squash (peeled), or 1 unpeeled butternut squash

175g pearl barley

Juice and zest of 1 orange

3 tbsp olive oil

½ red onion, sliced thinly

4 tbsp red wine vinegar

2 handfuls rocket

1 bunch flat-leaf parsley (small), chopped. Set aside several leaves for serving.

1 bunch mint (small), chopped. Set aside several leaves for serving.

Directions:

For 20 to 25 minutes or until just tender, boil the barley. Drain. Meanwhile, heat the oven to 200°C. When using butternut, slice into thick rounds. You may also cut the squash into thin wedges. Remove the seeds. Toss with the orange zest, 1 tbsp oil, and seasoning. Place the squash rounds or wedges on a baking tray.

Spread them out, and roast for 40 minutes until tender and golden, turning the squash halfway through cooking. Set aside. Mix the vinegar, orange juice, and the rest of the oil with the barley. Season accordingly. Stir in the chopped herbs and onion. Arrange them on a platter with the rocket, squash, and the remaining parsley and mint leaves.

Serves: 6   **Prep Time:40 mins.**   **Cooking Time:40 mins.**

Calories:226   **Protein:5g**   **Carbs:40g**   **Fat:6g**

106. Chicken, Tomato, and Bean Soup

Ingredients:

1 onion, chopped

1 tbsp. olive oil

1 carrot, chopped

1 zucchini, chopped

2 stalks celery, chopped

410g four-bean mix, drained and rinsed

4 cups chicken stock

300g chicken thighs (skinless, boneless, sliced, and trimmed)

1 bay leaf

1 tsp oregano, dried

150g baby spinach leaves, dried

1 lemon zest (grated), optional

Directions:

In a large saucepan on medium flame, heat the oil. Add the onion and cook for 10 minutes, or until golden and soft. Add the celery and carrot and cook until soft or for 5 minutes. Mix in the tomatoes, zucchini, four-bean mix, 1 cup water, chicken, and chicken stock. Add the oregano, bay leaf, and lemon zest. Simmer the soup mixture for 20 minutes, or until the chicken is thoroughly cooked and the vegetables become tender. Add the chopped spinach and cook for 2 more minutes, or until the leaves are wilted.

Serves: 4	**Prep Time:15 mins.**	**Cooking Time:40 mins.**
Calories:352	**Protein:23g**	**Carbs:20g**	**Fat:9g**

107. Caraway and Roasted Carrot Soup

Ingredients:

1 kg carrots

1 onion, chopped finely

1 tbsp olive oil

2 cloves garlic, chopped

4 cups vegetable stock, reduced salt

1 ½ tbsp caraway seeds, add more to serve

4 slices whole grain bread, for serving

Ground black pepper, to taste

Directions:

Preheat oven to 350°F (180°C). Use parchment paper to line a baking tray. Peel the carrots and cut them into lengthwise quarters. Put the carrot portions on the tray and roast until they're lightly browned and tender, or for 45 minutes. In a large saucepan, heat the oil. For 4 minutes over medium heat, and cook onions until translucent. Add garlic and caraway seeds then cook for one more minute. Add in the carrots, 1 cup (250ml) water, and stock. Puree the soup using a stick blender. Boil the soup. Reduce the heat and simmer the soup for 5 more minutes. Use ground pepper to season the soup. Ladle the soup into bowls and garnish with more caraway seeds. Serve together with the whole grain bread slices.

Serves: 4	**Prep Time:20 mins.**	**Cooking Time:55 mins.**
Calories:153	**Protein:4g**	**Carbs:21g**	**Fat:6g**

108. Vegetable and Duck Soup

Ingredients:

350g duck breast (with the fat trimmed off), chopped

1 tbsp oil

2 cloves garlic, crushed

1 leek, white part

2 stalks celery, sliced thinly

1 carrot, sliced and halved

2 cups chicken stock

410g tomatoes, diced

1 bay leaf

¼ cabbage, shredded

1 zucchini, sliced and halved

2 tbsp parsley (fresh), chopped

In a large saucepan or stock pot on high, heat half of the oil. In batches, cook the duck until browned, or for 2 to 3 minutes. Stir often. Set aside the cooked duck. In the pot, heat the rest of the oil. On low heat, cook the garlic and leek until soft, or for 3 to 5 minutes. Add the celery and carrot to the pot. Add the tomatoes, duck, bay leaf, 2 cups water, and stock. Boil the mixture, and then reduce the heat. Simmer for one hour, or until the vegetables and duck are tender. If the soup is too thick, add more water. Stir in the cabbage and zucchini, and cook for 5 minutes longer, or until the vegetables become tender. Remove the bay leaf. Use the chopped parsley to sprinkle the soup. Ladle into bowls. Serve and enjoy.

Serves: 4   **Prep Time:20 mins.**   **Cooking Time: 1 hr. 15 mins.**

Calories:206   **Protein:22g**   **Carbs:10g**   **Fat:9g**

109. Leek Soup with Flatbread and Oysters

Ingredients:

Leek Soup and Oysters:
2 tbsp. olive oil
1 3/4lb leeks, whole
2 cups chicken stock
300g potatoes (roughly diced), unpeeled
12 oysters, fresh
2 tbsp. fresh chives, snipped

Black pepper (ground), to taste
Flatbreads:
2 tsp yeast, dry
1/3 cup poppy seeds
¾ cup flour (plain), whole meal
2 tbsp olive oil

Directions:

Make the flatbreads by pouring 85ml lukewarm water in a bowl. Sprinkle it with the yeast and leave on for several minutes for the yeast to rehydrate. Put in the flour, and thoroughly mix to form a soft dough. Kneed the seeds into the dough until they're fully incorporated and the dough has become a sticky, smooth ball. Allow the dough to rest.

Preheat oven to 480°F (250°C). Use parchment or baking paper to line a baking tray. Cut the leeks lengthwise. Wash the leeks well and slice thinly the green and white parts. Discard the rest of the leeks. In a large saucepan, heat the olive oil and, over low heat, cook the leeks until soft or for 5 minutes. Add the stock and potatoes to the pan, and simmer the mixture until the potatoes are softened, or for 15 minutes.

Meanwhile, divide the flatbread into four portions, and roll each part into a ball. Use flour to dust a rolling pin and work surface. Roll each flatbread ball, as thin as you can, into a long oval. Put the flat ovals on prepared baking tray. Space them apart and brush each oval with oil. Bake until golden and crisp or for 10 to 15 minutes.

Let to soup to slightly cool. Transfer to a food processor or blender and blend until the soup contents are smooth. Use stock, milk, or water to dilute the soup. Dilute until you achieve the right consistency. Divide the soup mixture into four bowls. Top each bowl with three oysters. Sprinkle with cracked black pepper and chives. Serve the soup with the flatbreads.

Serves: 4   **Prep Time:20 mins.**   **Cooking Time:25 mins.**
Calories:474   **Protein:20g**   **Carbs:39g**   **Fat:27g**

110. Miso Soup with Ginger and Edamame

Ingredients:

1 carrot, sliced thinly

4 spring onions, sliced diagonally and thinly

1 daikon, sliced thinly

2 inches peeled ginger (fresh), julienned

6 shiitake mushrooms (dried), cut into small pieces

2 tbsp. shiro miso

150g firm tofu (silken), cubed

180g edamame soybeans, shelled

Directions:

In a large saucepan, add 1.25 liters (5 cups) water. Add the carrot, spring onions, dried mushrooms, daikon, and ginger. Boil, and then reduce heat. Simmer the soup mixture for 15 minutes. Spoon out about 2 tablespoons of the soup and add it to the miso. Stir back the miso into the pot.

Do not boil the soup. Add the tofu and edamame, and cook further for 5 minutes, or until the edamame is tender and bright green. Among 4 bowls, divide the vegetables and tofu. Ladle the hot stock into the bowls. Serve hot and enjoy.

Serves: 4	Prep Time:10 mins.		Cooking Time:25 mins.
Calories:148	Protein:10g	Carbs:20g	Fat:4g

111. Arugula, Beet, And Chickpea Salad with Lemon-Chia Dressing

Ingredients:

1 tablespoon fresh lemon juice

2 teaspoon olive oil

½ teaspoon honey

2 teaspoon chia seeds

¼ teaspoon Dijon mustard

Pinch of salt

1 cup chickpeas, rinse and drain excess water

1 cup sliced steamed or roasted beets

1 cup arugula

1 tablespoon chopped fresh dill

2 tablespoons nutritional yeast

Directions:

Place olive oil, lemon juice, Dijon mustard, salt, honey and chia seeds in a bowl. Whisk well. Place chickpeas, beets, arugula, dill and nutritional yeast in a bowl. Toss together. Pour the dressing and toss to coat everything well. Serve.

Serves: 1	Prep Time:20 mins.		Cooking Time: 0 mins.
Calories:453	Protein:19g	Carbs:57g	Fat:19g

112. Grapefruit, Toasted Hazelnut, and Raw Kale Salad

Ingredients:

2 pieces of whole pink grapefruit

1/4 cup fresh lemon juice

1/2 small red onion, sliced thinly, divided

1/2 cup plain fat-free yogurt

1/2 teaspoon salt

2 tablespoons extra-virgin olive oil

1/4 teaspoon black pepper

1/3 cup chopped toasted hazelnuts

8 ounces lacinato kale or baby kale leaves, sliced very thinly

Directions:

Peel the grapefruit and separate into segments. Reserve 3 tablespoons of the grapefruit juice. Place in a large bowl. Place the segments in a separate bowl. Add lemon juice to the bowl with grapefruit juice. Add oil and yogurt into the juice mixture. Season with pepper and salt. Whisk the dressing well. Drizzle the dressing over the kale and toss well. Add onions, hazelnuts and grapefruit. Give the salad another quick toss. Serve immediately.

Serves: 4   **Prep Time:20 mins.**   **Cooking Time: 0 mins.**

Calories:184   **Protein:5g**   **Carbs:18g**   **Fat:11.6g**

113. Roasted Tomato and Red Bell Pepper Soup

Ingredients:

8 plum tomatoes (large), cut in half lengthwise

4 red bell peppers (large)

4 cloves garlic (large), unpeeled

1 red onion, sliced into 6 wedges

3 cups vegetable stock

1 ½ tbsp olive oil

16 sage leaves, fresh

2 tsp sage (fresh), chopped finely

Ground black pepper, to taste

Directions:

Preheat oven to 375°F (190°C). Use parchment paper to line two baking trays. On one tray, put the whole capsicum peppers. On the second tray, arrange tomatoes, with the cut-side up. Bake trays with vegetables for 20 minutes.

Add garlic and onion to the trays. Use 2 tablespoons olive oil to drizzle the onion. Bake further for 40 minutes, turning the peppers once, until the onions are tender and the tomatoes and capsicums are softened. Set aside to cool.

Peel the peppers, discarding the white membrane and seeds. Also peel the tomatoes. In a food processor, place the tomato flesh, capsicum, and onion. Extract the garlic's pulp from the seeds and add into the food processor. Puree the vegetables until you get a smooth consistency. Place the vegetable puree in a saucepan. Add the chopped sage and stock. Heat until the soup simmers.

On medium heat in a small frying pan, heat the remaining 1 tablespoon of olive oil. Put in the whole sage and cook until crisp. Drain the crisped sage on paper towels. Set the oil aside and slightly cool. Ladle the soup into bowls and top with the crisp sage leaves. Drizzle the soup with the reserved oil, and sprinkle each serving with ground black pepper.

Serves: 4   **Prep Time:20 mins.**   **Cooking Time: 1 hr. 15 mins.**

Calories:157   **Protein:6g**   **Carbs:14g**   **Fat:9g**

114.   *Turkey, Cauliflower, and Kale Soup*

Ingredients:

4 shallots, chopped
1 lb turkey, ground
3 carrots, sliced
1 can (15 oz) tomatoes, diced
1 bell pepper, cut to pieces
1 ½ cups cauliflower, chopped

5 cups chicken stock
2 tbsp coconut oil
4 cups kale (chopped coarsely), ribs removed
Ground black pepper
Sea salt

Directions:

In a saucepan on medium-high, melt the coconut oil. Add the carrots, shallots, bell pepper, and cauliflower. Sauté for 8 to 10 minutes or until the vegetables are softened slightly. Stir frequently. Add the turkey to the mixture and cook for 6 to 8 minutes, or until the meat is thoroughly cooked. Add the diced tomatoes and chicken stock. Season with pepper and salt. Boil the soup and add in the kale. Reduce the heat and simmer the soup on low for 15 minutes. Cover the pan. Serve and enjoy.

Serves: 4   **Prep Time:25 mins.**   **Cooking Time:45 mins.**
Calories:167   **Protein:37g**   **Carbs:28g**   **Fat:20g**

115. Citrus Salad with Crispy Quinoa

Ingredients:

Dressing:

3 tablespoons olive oil

1 tablespoon honey

2 tablespoons fresh lime juice

1/2 teaspoon salt

Salad:

1 pitted avocado, peeled, then diced

1/2 cup uncooked quinoa

2 peeled oranges, diced

5 cups spring lettuce mix

1/2 cup chopped scallions, both green and white parts

Directions:

Place all the ingredients for the dressing in a glass jar with a tight lid. Close the lid tightly and shake the jar to mix the dressing well. An immersion blender may also be used for mixing. Follow the package instructions about how to cook the quinoa. Set aside when cooked. Set the broiler heat setting to heat. Position the rack on the top third level.

Place the quinoa in a baking sheet with a rim. Spread into an even layer. Place the quinoa inside the broiler to toast. Stir occasionally. Check the quinoa frequently to see if it has started to turn crisp. The edges should turn golden brown. This may take around 10 to 12 minutes. Remove the quinoa from the broiler and set aside to cool.

Put the lettuce leaves in a large salad or mixing bowl. Put the scallions, avocado, cooled toasted quinoa and oranges as well. Shake or mix the dressing once more. Pour over the salad. Toss the salad until everything has been coated well with the dressing. Serve immediately.

Serves: 4	Prep Time:15 mins.		Cooking Time: 12 mins.
Calories:308	Protein:5g	Carbs:33g	Fat:19g

116. *Brussels Sprout and Apple Salad*

Ingredients:

1 apple, julienned

2 cups shredded Brussels sprouts

2-3 tablespoons extra virgin olive oil

Juice from half a lemon

¼ cup pine nuts

Salt and pepper to taste

Directions:

Place apple, Brussel sprouts, lemon juice and olive oil in a salad bowl. Season with some ground black pepper and a small amount of salt to taste. Toss. Transfer to a serving plate. Sprinkle with pine nuts and serve.

Serves: 2-4   **Prep Time:10 mins.**   **Cooking Time: 0 mins.**

Calories:324   **Protein:5.7g**   **Carbs:24g**   **Fat:26g**

117. *Greek Lentil Soup with Toasted Pita*

Ingredients:

1 tablespoon olive oil

2 carrots, remove and discard the peel, slice into smaller pieces

2 celery stalks, sliced into smaller pieces

2 garlic cloves, minced

1 onion

2 teaspoons dried oregano

1/2 teaspoon pepper

1/2 teaspoon salt

1 cup dry lentils

8 cups water

2 tablespoons freshly squeezed lemon juice

4 whole-grain pitas, each piece sliced into 4 triangles, toast

Directions:

Pour some oil into a large Dutch oven on medium heat. When oil is hot, add garlic, oregano, onion, carrot and celery. Season with pepper and salt. Cook for about 5 minutes. Add lentils. Pour water. Partially cover the Dutch oven and allow the soup to simmer for about 15 minutes. Take a potato masher or a hand blender to puree the soup until it becomes thick and semi-smooth. A few chunks will be fine. Stir a little before turning off the heat. Drizzle the lemon juice over the soup. Ladle into bowls and serve with the toasted pita.

Serves: 4   **Prep Time:15 mins.**   **Cooking Time:20 mins.**

Calories:370   **Protein:19g**   **Carbs:65g**   **Fat:6g**

118. Mexican Superfood Cabbage Soup

Ingredients:

2 tablespoons extra-virgin olive oil

1 cup chopped carrot

2 cups chopped onions

1 cup chopped celery

4 large cloves garlic, minced

1 cup chopped green bell pepper

8 cups sliced cabbage

1 tablespoon chipotle chilis in adobo sauce, minced

1 tablespoon tomato paste

½ teaspoon ground coriander

1 teaspoon ground cumin

4 cups water

4 cups low-sodium chicken broth or vegetable broth

2 15-ounce cans low-sodium black or pinto beans, rinsed

¾ teaspoon salt

2 tablespoons lime juice

½ cup chopped fresh cilantro, add more for serving

Garnish:

nonfat plain Greek yogurt

crumbled queso fresco

diced avocado

Directions:

Put oil in a large, deep soup pot. Heat over a stove set on medium heat setting. Put celery, carrots, bell peppers, garlic and onions. Frequently stir while cooking until vegetables start to soften. Put the cabbage in and cook for 10 more minutes until it softens. Add coriander, chipotle, tomato paste and cumin. Stir and cook for another minute. Add salt, beans and water. Cover the pot and allow to boil. Lower heat setting to a simmer. Simmer partially covered until the vegetables turn tender. Turn off the heat. Stir in the lime juice and cilantro. Serve with the garnishes.

Serves: 8   **Prep Time:20 mins.**   **Cooking Time:25 mins.**

Calories:174   **Protein:7g**   **Carbs:28g**   **Fat:4g**

119. Detox Superfood Vegetable Soup

Ingredients:

1 tablespoon olive oil

1 large peeled carrot, chopped

1 medium size yellow onion, diced

1 red bell pepper, sliced

2 stalks celery, chopped

4 cloves garlic, minced

1 28-ounce can dice tomatoes

4 cups stemmed kale, chopped

2 cups trimmed green beans, chopped

4 cups vegetable stock

1 teaspoon dried basil

1 1/2 teaspoon dried oregano

1/2 teaspoon dried thyme

1/2 teaspoon black pepper

1 teaspoon salt

2 tablespoons chopped fresh parsley

Directions

Place a large pot over a stove set to medium high heat. Pour the olive oil into the pan and allow to heat up. Put celery, carrots and onions. Cook the vegetables until the onions turn translucent. Add bell pepper and garlic. Cook for another minute. Put the green beans. Cook for 1 more minute. Add the spices and the tomatoes. Pour the vegetable stock in. Stir the soup then allow to boil. Reduce the heat to a simmer. Let the soup simmer uncovered for about 25 minutes over medium low heat setting. Put the kale into the soup. Cook the soup for another 5 minutes. Turn the heat off and add the fresh parsley. Ladle into soup bowls. Serve warm.

Serves: 6	Prep Time:15 mins.		Cooking Time:37 mins.
Calories:115	Protein:4.6g	Carbs:20.5g	Fat:2.8g

120. Superfood Salmon Salad

Ingredients

100 g couscous

2 salmon fillets

1 tablespoon olive oil

200 g sprouting broccoli, removed larger stalks then roughly shred the rest

seeds from half of a pomegranate

juice from 1 piece of lemon

2 handfuls watercress

small handful pumpkin seeds

extra olive oil and lemon wedges, for serving

Directions

Mix 1 teaspoon of oil and couscous. Boil water and pour it over the couscous. Pour enough to cover the couscous by 1 centimeter. Set this aside. Blanch the broccoli until it turns bright green and tender. Drain and rinse immediately with cold water. Steam the salmon until opaque and flaky, about 3 minutes. Transfer to a plate. Mix the rest of the lemon juice and the oil. Put pumpkin seeds, broccoli and pomegranate seeds into the bowl with the couscous. Pour the lemon dressing over the couscous mixture. Chop watercress roughly and put in the bowl. Toss everything to mix. Transfer to a plate. Place the salmon on top of the couscous and lemon wedges on the side. Drizzle with some olive oil and serve.

Serves: 2	Prep Time:10 mins.	Cooking Time: 10 mins.

Calories:320   **Protein:30g**   **Carbs:30g**   **Fat:10g**

121. Winter Squash and Bison Stew

Ingredients

1 medium winter squash

1 Tbs extra virgin olive oil

1 sweet onion

6 cloves garlic

2 celery stalks

2 carrots

3 cups broccoli

2 sprigs fresh rosemary

2 sprigs fresh thyme

1 bay leaf

1 can garbanzo beans

2 Tbs extra virgin olive oil

1-pound bison stew meat

1/2 tsp chili powder

1/2 tsp cumin

2 quarts chicken broth

2 Tbs apple cider vinegar

Directions

Preheat oven to 350 degrees. Cut squash in half and remove seeds. Spread oil on cut sides. Place cut side down in baking dish, and bake forty-five minutes to an hour, until squash is soft. While squash is baking, prep remainder of the ingredients. When squash is finished, scoop out flesh and cut into bite-sized chunks. Peel and chop onion. Finely chop garlic. Chop celery and carrots. Chop broccoli crowns, and peel and chop broccoli stems. Place rosemary, thyme, and bay leaf in an herb bag. Rinse and drain beans. Sauté onions over medium heat, with extra virgin olive oil, in a large dutch oven or soup pot, until soft. Add bison and continue to cook, stirring frequently, until browned on all sides. Add garlic, celery, carrots, spices, broth, beans, and apple cider vinegar. Bring to a boil, then reduce heat. Add herb bag and simmer for ten minutes. Add broccoli and squash and cook for a further ten minutes. Remove herb bag and ladle stew into bowls. Enjoy!

Serves: 4   **Prep Time:10 mins.**   **Cooking Time:1 hr.**

Calories: 424.5   **Protein: 30.8g**   **Carbs: 58.3g**   **Fat: 7.9g**

122. Kale & Quinoa Salad with Lemon Vinaigrette

Ingredients

2 cups cooked quinoa

3 cups Tuscan kale, remove ribs then finely chop

1 1/2 cup cooked edamame beans, cooled

1/2 red onion, diced

1 cup sliced grape tomatoes

1 pitted avocado, diced

1 pitted mango, diced

2 tablespoon pumpkin seeds or toasted almonds, if desired

For lemon vinaigrette

1/4 cup fresh squeezed lemon juice

2 tablespoons olive oil

1 teaspoon sugar

1 clove garlic, minced

1 large basil leaf, chopped

fresh ground pepper, to taste

1/8 teaspoon salt

Directions

To make the dressing, pour the lemon juice and oil in a food processor. Add the salt, basil, garlic and sugar. Pulse everything to create a smooth and evenly mixed dressing. Set aside. Put kale, edamame and quinoa in a mixing bowl. Pour the dressing over the quinoa mixture. Toss until all the ingredients are coated with the vinaigrette. Chill for about 20 to 30 minutes. Toss the salad again. Add the avocado, mango, onion and tomato. Serve with a garnish of pumpkin seeds or toasted almonds.

Serves: 4   Prep Time:35 mins.   Cooking Time:0 mins.

Calories:390   Protein:13.9g   Carbs:47.7g   Fat:17.4g

123. Kale Salad

Ingredients

4 ounces mixed baby greens or baby spinach leaves

1 bunch of de-stemmed lacinato kale, sliced into bite-size pieces

1 cup chopped red cabbage

2 peeled carrots, sliced into thin ribbons

1 cup cooked black beans

4 small caps Portobello mushrooms, slice lengthwise

1/2 red bell pepper, sliced

1 bunch Brussels sprouts, trim and discard ends then slice the rest into quarters

2-3 teaspoons avocado or olive oil

1/4 cup raw sunflower seeds

1 avocado, slice

Balsamic dressing

1/4 cup balsamic vinegar

2 tablespoons olive oil

Juice from 1/2 of a lemon

2 tablespoons maple syrup

1 teaspoon Dijon mustard

1 teaspoon minced garlic

1/2 teaspoon ground pepper

1/2 teaspoon salt

Directions

Place the ingredients for the dressing in a mixing bowl and whisk them together until smooth. Put the mushrooms with the dressing. Mix to coat well. Set aside to marinate for 1 hour to overnight. Prepare the oven to 375F. Coat the Brussels sprouts with 2 to 3 teaspoons of oil. Season with pepper and salt. Arrange the Brussels sprouts in a single layer on a baking sheet. Roast in the preheated oven for 40 to 45 minutes until browned and tender. Turn occasionally during the roasting. Place the marinated mushrooms together with the marinade in a deep bowl. Add all the other salad ingredients into the mushrooms. Stir to coat everything evenly. Let the salad stand for a few minutes before serving. This will allow all the flavors to meld. Serve salad topped with an avocado slice and sprinkled with some sunflower seeds.

Serves: 3   Prep Time: 1 hr. 15 mins.   Cooking Time:55 mins.
Calories:484   Protein:16g   Carbs:55g   Fat:26g

124. Turmeric Egg Soup

Ingredients:

1 tablespoon olive oil

1 cup water

1 egg

1 teaspoon fresh, crushed garlic

1 teaspoon fresh ginger

½ teaspoon turmeric

Directions:

Heat oil and sauté garlic and ginger. Add turmeric and fry for approximately two minutes. Break in the egg and sauté until thoroughly cooked. Add water and heat to boil, add salt to taste, cover and simmer for approximately 20 minutes.

Serves: 2   **Prep Time:10 mins.**   **Cooking Time:45 mins.**

Calories: 237   **Protein: 13g**   **Carbs: 40g**   **Fat: 5g**

125. Butternut Squash Soup with Coconut and Ginger

Ingredients

2 large butternut squash

3 Tbs coconut oil

Himalayan salt to taste

Fresh ground black pepper to taste

1 medium yellow onion, finely chopped

1 rib celery, diced

2 Tbs fresh ginger

1 cup chard

1 cup cilantro

1 cup coconut flakes

1 tsp turmeric

 tsp curry powder

1/2 cup white wine

6 cups chicken broth

1 can unsweetened coconut milk

1 fresh thyme sprig

Directions

Preheat oven to 350 degrees. Cut squash in half lengthwise. Spread cut sides with 2 tablespoons coconut oil; sprinkle liberally with salt and pepper. Cover cut sides with foil, and bake until tender, about an hour and a half. When cool enough to handle, scoop out flesh. While squash is cooking, prepare remainder of ingredients. Finely chop onion. Dice celery. Peel and finely mince or grate ginger. Chop chard and cilantro. Toast coconut flakes in a dry skillet over medium heat, stirring frequently. In a large soup pot, melt remaining coconut oil over medium heat. Add onions, celery, ginger, turmeric, and curry powder; cook, stirring frequently, until onions are translucent. Add wine and cook until nearly evaporated. Add chard and cook until wilted. Mix in squash and remove from heat. Allow to cool slightly, and puree with a countertop or immersion blender. Return to soup pot; add broth and coconut milk. Mix well. Add thyme sprig and simmer over medium-low heat for twenty minutes or until you're ready to eat! Remember to remove the thyme sprig before serving. Sprinkle with coconut flakes and cilantro to serve.

Serves: 6   **Prep Time:40 mins.**   **Cooking Time:1 hr. 30 mins.**

Calories: 100   **Protein: 2g**   **Carbs: 20g**   **Fat: 2.5g**

126. *Broccoli and Almond Soup*

Ingredients

1/2 cup slivered almonds

1 medium yellow onion

3 ribs celery

2 Tbs fresh parsley

2 cloves garlic

2 heads broccoli

1 Tbs olive oil

1 Tbs tamari

1 Tbs fresh thyme

1 Tbs fresh marjoram

1 tsp Himalayan salt

1 tsp black pepper

2 cups chicken stock

3 Tbs almond butter

1 can coconut milk

Directions

Toast almonds in a dry skillet over medium heat; set aside. Chop onions, celery, and parsley. Peel and press or finely chop garlic. Chop broccoli; peel and chop stems as well. In a dutch oven or soup pot, sauté onion, garlic, tamari, thyme, marjoram, salt, and pepper in olive oil over medium heat until onions are soft. Add broccoli and celery, and continue to cook, stirring frequently, for five to seven minutes. Add stock and almond butter, increase heat, and bring to a boil. Reduce heat and simmer until broccoli is nearly done, being careful not to overcook. Remove from heat; allow to cool slightly. Using an immersion or countertop blender, puree the soup and stir in coconut milk. Serve soup garnished with parsley.

Serves: 4   **Prep Time:10 mins.**   **Cooking Time:50 mins.**

Calories: 140   **Protein: 6.1g**   **Carbs: 12.1g**   **Fat: 8.2g**

127. Beet Soup

Ingredients

6 large beets
2 finely chopped shallots
1/2-inch fresh ginger, grated
Juice of two limes
1 tsp ground cumin

1 tsp coconut oil
1-quart chicken or vegetable stock
1 15-oz. can coconut milk
2 Tbs cilantro

Directions

To roast beets, preheat oven to 350 degrees. Wash beets gently to leave skin in place. Trim, leaving an inch or so of the stem and taproot. Place in a baking dish with about ½ cup water, cover, and bake until soft, about forty-five minutes. Allow to cool slightly, rub skin off, and dice. Peel and finely chop shallots. Grate ginger. Juice limes. Sauté shallots, cumin, and ginger in coconut oil in a large soup pot over medium heat. When shallots are soft, add beets and stock. Bring to a boil, then reduce heat and simmer five minutes. Let cool slightly and use a blender to puree. Stir in coconut milk and lime juice. Ladle into bowls; garnish with cilantro.

Serves: 4   Prep Time:10 mins.   Cooking Time:45 mins.
Calories: 102.9   Protein: 5.6g   Carbs: 17.9g   Fat: 1.5g

128. *Black Bean and Sweet Potato Soup*

Ingredients

4 cups black beans	2 cups water
1/2 cup shallot	1 tsp turmeric
2 cloves garlic	2 tsp cumin
2 large sweet potatoes	1 Tbs chili powder
1 cup red cabbage	1 tsp ground coriander
1 lime	1 tsp Himalayan salt
1 Tbs coconut oil	1/2 tsp black pepper
1 Tbs pumpkin seeds	1 avocado
1-quart chicken or vegetable broth	½ cup cilantro

Directions

If you're using dried beans, soak half a pound overnight. Otherwise, drain and rinse two cans of beans. Peel and chop the shallot, garlic, and sweet potatoes. Chop the cabbage. Juice the lime. In a large soup pot, heat the coconut oil over medium heat. Add in the shallot, garlic, and pumpkin seeds, and cook until tender, stirring frequently. Stir in sweet potato. Cook for five minutes. Add in broth, water, lime juice, black beans, and red cabbage. Stir well. Add the turmeric, cumin, chili powder, and coriander. Stir. Bring to a boil, then reduce heat and simmer on medium-low heat until sweet potatoes are soft, about thirty minutes. Remove 2 cups of soup; blend with a countertop or immersion blender. Return to soup pot, stir in salt and pepper. Peel and cube avocado, chop cilantro. Ladle soup into bowls, and sprinkle with avocado cubes and cilantro.

Serves: 4   **Prep Time:15 mins.**   **Cooking Time: 1 hr.**

Calories: 230.7   **Protein: 12g**   **Carbs: 45.8g**   **Fat: 3.4g**

129. *Restorative Chicken Soup*

Ingredients

3 quarts chicken broth

1 whole chicken

1 celery root, peeled and coarsely chopped

1 coarsely chopped yellow onion

1 coarsely chopped carrot

6 peeled garlic cloves

10 whole black peppercorns

10 thyme sprigs

6 carrots

3 parsnips

1/4 cup brown mustard

1/2 tsp salt

1/2 tsp pepper

1 zucchini

1 tsp thyme

Directions

In a large soup pot, combine broth, chicken, celery root, onion, 1 coarsely chopped carrot, garlic, peppercorns, and thyme sprigs. Bring to a boil, then reduce heat and simmer until chicken is cooked, about 1½ hours. Transfer chicken to a platter and let cool. Meanwhile, prepare the rest of the dish. Debone the chicken when cool. Strain the broth and return it to the pot. Discard (or compost) the veggies. Bring to a boil over high heat, skimming as necessary, until reduced to 6 cups, about fifteen minutes. Cover and keep hot. Peel parsnips.

Dice carrots and parsnips. In a medium saucepan, bring carrots and parsnips to a boil, then reduce heat and simmer until tender. Drain and set aside. You may wish to cook the carrots and parsnips separately to preserve their individual flavors. Combine carrots, parsnips, deboned chicken and 1 cup of broth in a large pot over medium-high heat; cover. Remove from heat when warm. Stir mustard, salt, and pepper into broth. Chop zucchini into matchsticks; chop thyme. Divide chicken and vegetables among bowls; add zucchini. Sprinkle with thyme, then ladle enough hot broth to cover.

Serves: 6   **Prep Time:15 mins.**   **Cooking Time: 2 hrs. 15 mins.**

Calories: 157   **Protein: 22g**   **Carbs: 16g**   **Fat: 1g**

130.   Coconut Ginger Salmon Soup

Ingredients

1-pound wild salmon, skinned, deboned and cubed

1 tsp Himalayan salt

3 chopped shallots

1 Tbs coconut oil

4 cups chicken stock

2 cans coconut milk

1-inch grated ginger

2 stalks fresh lemon grass

1/2 tsp red curry paste

1/2 tsp fish sauce

1 tsp Himalayan salt

4 oz. rice noodles

1 bunch chopped baby bok choy

1 lime, cut into wedges

2 Tbs chopped cilantro

Directions

Season the salmon to taste with salt. Refrigerate for thirty minutes while preparing the soup. In a stock pot, add shallots and coconut oil then sauté until translucent. Add salt, fish sauce, curry, lemon grass, coconut milk and stock. Allow to boil on medium heat then continue to cook for about 20 minutes. Decrease heat to low and simmer another five minutes. Raise the heat back to a medium flame then add salmon and allow to simmer for another 5 minutes. Add rice noodles and baby bok choy and continue to simmer until the noodles are cooked (about 5 minutes). Ladle into bowls, garnish with cilantro and lime wedges.

Serves: 4   **Prep Time:10 mins.**   **Cooking Time:20 mins.**

Calories: 210.2   **Protein: 26.9g**   **Carbs: 2.4g**   **Fat: 8.5g**

131. *Quinoa Salad with Black Beans*

Ingredients

1½ cups quinoa

1 can black beans

3 cups chicken broth

1 avocado, peeled and chopped

2 carrots, grated

3 dates, chopped

1/2 cup cilantro, chopped

2½ limes, juiced

1½ Tbs apple cider vinegar

1 tsp cumin, or more to taste

1/3 cup extra virgin olive oil

1/4 tsp salt

Directions

Rinse and drain quinoa and beans. Add broth to a saucepan, and allow to boil, add quinoa, cover, and simmer on low heat until all the quinoa is tender and the liquid is fully absorbed (about 15 minutes). Allow to cool. In a bowl, combine salt, oil, cumin, vinegar and lime juice then whisk. In another bowl, mix cilantro, dates, carrots, avocado, beans and quinoa. Add dressing and gently toss. Serve and enjoy!

Serves: 4   **Prep Time:15 mins.**   **Cooking Time:15 mins.**

Calories: 370.7   **Protein: 10.6g**   **Carbs: 55.1g**   **Fat: 13.2g**

132. *Celery Root Soup*

Ingredients

1/2 cup pumpkin seeds

1 tsp salt

1 chopped medium onion

1 Tbs chopped fresh thyme

1 peeled and chopped celery root

2 peeled and sliced parsnips

1 sliced lemon

 Tbs olive oil

1/2 tsp ground pepper

1 tsp turmeric

6 cups vegetable or chicken stock

Directions

Toast pumpkin seeds in a dry skillet over medium heat. Toss with 1/2 teaspoon salt and set aside. Dice onion and thyme. Peel and dice celery root and parsnips. Slice lemon into wedges. In a soup pot, sauté onion in olive oil over medium heat until soft. Add remainder of salt, pepper, turmeric, thyme, celery root, parsnips, and stock. Bring to a boil, then reduce heat and simmer until vegetables are soft, about twenty minutes. Remove from heat, let cool slightly, and puree with an immersion or countertop blender. Serve with a squeeze of lemon juice and garnished with toasted pumpkin seeds.

Serves: 4   **Prep Time:15 mins.**   **Cooking Time:40 mins.**

Calories: 73.9   **Protein: 1.7g**   **Carbs: 8.7g**   **Fat: 2.6g**

133.   Coconut Carrot Soup

Ingredients

2 Tbs coconut oil

1 chopped large shallot

2 Tbs chopped fresh ginger

1½ tsp curry powder

4 cups chicken or vegetable broth

5 chopped medium carrots

2 cups cubed sweet potatoes

1 can (13.5 oz.) unsweetened coconut milk

Himalayan salt to taste

Black pepper to taste

2 Tbs chopped cilantro

1 lime, cut into wedges

Directions

In a soup pot, heat oil over medium heat. Add shallot and a splash of broth, and sauté about two minutes. Add ginger and sauté another two minutes. Add curry powder and stir until fragrant. Add remaining broth, carrots, and sweet potatoes, and simmer on medium-high heat until vegetables are tender (about fifteen minutes). Add coconut milk, and salt and pepper to taste. Use an immersion blender or blend in batches, making sure blender is not more than half full. Return to soup pot and reheat. Serve piping hot in bowls garnished with cilantro and fresh lime wedges.

Serves: 4   **Prep Time:15 mins.**   **Cooking Time:30 mins.**

Calories: 163.8   **Protein: 3.4g**   **Carbs: 21g**   **Fat: 8.6g**

134. Sunshine Stew

Ingredients

1-inch piece ginger
3 cloves garlic
1 medium shallot
4 ounces split red lentils
1 small sweet potato
3 medium carrots
3 leaves kale
1 lime
2 Tbs coconut oil

2 tsp ground coriander
2 tsp ground cumin
1 Tbs red curry paste (optional)
1 Tbs turmeric
1 (13-oz.) can coconut milk
1-quart chicken stock
1 (15-oz.) can pumpkin puree
black pepper, to taste
Himalayan salt, to taste

Directions

Peel and grate ginger. Peel and press or mince garlic. Thinly slice shallot. Wash and drain lentils. Dice sweet potato. Chop carrots and kale. Slice lime into wedges. Heat coconut oil in a heavy stockpot. Sauté ginger, garlic, and shallot until shallot is translucent. Add coriander, cumin, red curry paste, and turmeric; continue to sauté a few more minutes. Add in coconut milk, chicken stock, and lentils. Increase heat, and bring to a boil for twenty minutes, stirring occasionally. Reduce heat to medium, add in sweet potato and carrots, and simmer for a further forty minutes, or until sweet potato is soft. Just before serving, stir in kale, salt, and pepper as needed. Ladle into bowls, and garnish with lime wedges.

Serves: 4   Prep Time:25 mins.   Cooking Time:50 mins.
Calories: 198   Protein: 4.2g   Carbs: 28.6g   Fat: 5.3g

135. Carrot and Black-Eyed Pea Salad

Ingredients

1/2 cup cashews
1 cup dried black-eyed peas
1 large garlic clove
1/2-inch ginger
1/2 cup extra virgin olive oil
Juice of 2 limes
1 tsp turmeric
1 Tbs maple syrup

1 tsp ground cumin
1/2 tsp Himalayan salt
1/8 tsp cayenne pepper
1/2 cup dried dates
4–6 carrots
1 bunch kale
1/3 cup fresh cilantro
1 avocado

Directions

Chop cashews and toast them in a dry skillet over medium-high heat, stirring frequently. Remove from heat and set aside. If using dried black-eyed peas, cook according to package directions to make 2 cups cooked beans. Drain, rinse, and set aside to cool. Substitute drained and rinsed canned beans if you prefer. Mince garlic and grate ginger. Whisk together, along with olive oil, lime juice, turmeric, maple syrup, cumin, salt, and cayenne pepper. Set aside. Chop dates into small pieces, being mindful of the pits. Shred enough carrots to make 1½ cups. Chop kale, including stems. Chop cilantro. Peel and dice avocado. In a medium bowl, combine the carrots, black-eyed peas, dried dates, cashews, kale, and cilantro. Mix in dressing and toss gently until everything is evenly coated. Toss in avocado. Serve immediately, or cover and refrigerate until ready to serve.

Serves: 4	Prep Time:45 mins.	Cooking Time:0 mins.	
Calories: 166	Protein: 4.2g	Carbs: 28.6g	Fat: 5.3g

136. Beet and Yogurt Salad

Ingredients

4 medium size beets

Extra virgin olive oil

1/4 cup shallots

4 garlic cloves

2 Tbs mint

2 Tbs cilantro

1½ Tbs sherry vinegar

1 tsp molasses

2 Tbs extra virgin olive oil

1/4 tsp mustard seeds

1/4 tsp cumin seeds

1/2 cup plain goat yogurt

1/4 tsp Himalayan salt

1/4 tsp freshly ground pepper

2 Tbs pine nuts

Directions

Remove greens from beets and set aside. Drizzle whole beets with extra virgin olive oil and roast in a foil packet at 350 degrees until tender, 25 to 60 minutes, depending on the size of the beets. Peel and chop into bite-sized pieces or slices. While beets are baking, prepare the rest of the ingredients. Peel and dice shallots. Peel and finely chop garlic. Chop mint, cilantro, and beet greens. Stir together the vinegar, molasses, olive oil, and salt and pepper to taste. Toss with the warm beets and marinate for 2 to 3 hours at room temperature or in the refrigerator.

Heat 2 tablespoons extra virgin olive oil over medium heat, add shallots and half the garlic. Sauté until onion is translucent. Add mustard seeds, stirring frequently. When they begin to pop, add the cumin seeds. Add in beet greens, and sauté for a few more minutes, stirring frequently. Mash the remainder of the garlic and salt. Stir into the yogurt. Add pepper. Drain the beets, saving some of the marinade to stir into the yogurt. Add beets to dressing and toss gently to coat. Make a bed of beet greens on the plates. Place the beets in the center of the greens and top with pine nuts, mint and cilantro.

Serves: 4   Prep Time:20 mins.   Cooking Time:1 hr.

Calories: 27.4   Protein: 2.4g   Carbs: 4.4g   Fat: 0.1g

137. Thai Chicken Salad

Ingredients

2 Thai chili peppers

2 cloves garlic

2 inches fresh ginger

1/2 cup cilantro

1/2 cup basil

1/2 cup red onion

1 cucumber

2 tomatoes

1-pound chicken

4 limes

1 head romaine lettuce

1/4 cup tamari

1/4 cup fish sauce

2 Tbs blackstrap molasses

1/2 tsp toasted sesame oil

1 Tbs sesame oil

Directions

Seed and chop chili peppers. Peel and roughly chop garlic and ginger. Chop cilantro. Cut basil into ribbons. Thinly slice onion crosswise. Slice cucumber and tomatoes. Cut chicken slices across the grain. Juice limes. Tear romaine leaves into bite-sized pieces. In a blender or food processor, pulse peppers, garlic, and ginger until finely chopped. Add tamari, fish sauce, molasses, cilantro, and lime juice; process until well combined. Separate 1/3 cup of mixture for salad dressing; set aside. Whisk reserved sauce with sesame oil to make salad dressing. In a large bowl, toss romaine, basil, onion, cucumber, and tomatoes with salad dressing. Heat oil in a large skillet over medium heat. Sauté chicken over medium-high heat for 1 minute per side, and toss with remaining sauce. Divide salad among dishes; top with chicken slices.

Serves: 4	Prep Time:10 mins.		Cooking Time:20 mins.
Calories: 281	Protein: 26g	Carbs: 40g	Fat: 8g

138. Sweet Potato Salad

Ingredients

1/2 cup frozen edamame

3 pounds sweet potatoes

1/2-inch ginger

1/2 lime

1/2 small red onion

3 stalks celery

1/4 cup fresh dill

2 tablespoons Dijon mustard

1/8 tsp cinnamon

1/4 tsp Himalayan salt

1/4 tsp black pepper

Directions

Thaw and shell edamame. Dice sweet potatoes. Grate ginger. Juice lime. Thinly slice onion and celery. Finely chop dill. In a medium saucepan with a steamer basket and 1 inch of water, steam sweet potatoes until tender, ten to fifteen minutes. Allow to cool. Whisk together lime juice, mustard, ginger, cinnamon, salt, and pepper. Combine onion, edamame, celery, and dill in a large bowl. Stir in sweet potatoes, and toss with dressing. Cover and refrigerate at least two, and up to twenty-four, hours.

Serves: 4	Prep Time:10 mins. + chilling time		Cooking Time:15 mins.
Calories: 177.5	Protein: 7.5g	Carbs: 37.4g	Fat:1g

139. Avocado and Watercress Salad

Ingredients

6 cups watercress
1 avocado
1/4 cup sweet onion
1 pomegranate
1/2 cup slivered almonds

1/4 cup rice vinegar
4 tsp tamari
1 tsp honey
3 Tbs extra virgin olive oil

Directions

Prepare the watercress by rinsing in cold water, then removing any yellowed or limp leaves and trimming excess stems. Peel and slice the avocado, finely slice the onion, and seed the pomegranate. Toast the almonds in a dry skillet over medium heat, stirring frequently. Whisk together vinegar, tamari, and honey until blended, then stir in oil. Toss watercress with enough dressing to coat, stir in onion, pomegranate seeds, and almonds. Divide watercress among plates, garnish with avocado slices.

Serves: 4   Prep Time:15 mins.   Cooking Time:0 mins.
Calories: 83   Protein: 1.4g   Carbs: 4.9g   Fat:7.1g

140. Spicy Salmon Slaw

Ingredients

Sprouted rice
1-pound red cabbage
1-pound carrots
1/2 cup fresh cilantro
3 limes
2 Tbs olive oil

Lime juice
1/2 tsp Himalayan salt
1/2 tsp ground pepper
1 tsp turmeric
1 tsp ginger
4 salmon filets

Directions

Cook rice according to package directions, enough for four servings. Shred cabbage. Coarsely grate carrot. Chop cilantro. Juice 2 limes. Cut another lime into wedges. Whisk oil, lime juice, salt, and pepper in a small bowl. In a large bowl, toss cabbage, carrots, and cilantro with dressing. Mix well and refrigerate until ready to serve. Stir turmeric and ginger together. Gently rub salmon with spice mixture. Grill six to eight minutes per side, or until salmon reaches desired temperature. Divide slaw among plates; serve with sliced salmon and rice.

Serves: 4   Prep Time:15 mins.   Cooking Time:45 mins.
Calories: 139.6   Protein: 15.4g   Carbs: 0.9g   Fat: 7.9g

Mind Diet Dessert Recipes

141. *Raspberry Soufflé*
Ingredients:

14 oz raspberries
½ cup confectioner's sugar
2 eggs, separated

1 tsp vanilla extract
1 ½ tbsp. pistachios, chopped finely
2 egg whites, extra

Preheat oven to 350°F (180°C). Slightly oil 6 ramekins (200ml). Sprinkle ½ teaspoon of the confectioner's sugar into every ramekin. In a food processor or blender, puree the raspberries. Use a sieve to take out the seeds. Measure out ¼ of the puree and reserve. Combine the rest of the puree with the egg yolks and the vanilla. In a dry, large bowl, use electric beaters to beat 4 egg whites until you form soft peaks. Slowly add the remaining sugar.

Beat after each sugar addition, until it has dissolved and the mix is glossy and thick. Stir a heaping spoonful of the egg whites into the egg yolk-raspberry mix. Use a large metal spoon to fold in gently the rest of the egg whites until the mixture is thoroughly combined and there are no lumps. Spoon the mixture into the ramekins, which you then put on a baking tray. Bake until the soufflés rise and are slightly golden, or for about 15 minutes. Immediately serve the soufflés, and top with the raspberry puree and the pistachios.

Serves: 6	**Prep Time:20 mins.**	**Cooking Time:15 mins.**
Calories:147	**Protein:5g**	**Carbs:24g**	**Fat:3g**

142. *Creamy Avocado Cups*
Ingredients

1 avocado
1 tablespoon reduced-fat sour cream or plain yogurt
1 tablespoon lime juice

1 tablespoon chopped fresh cilantro
1/4 teaspoon ground cumin
12 endive leaves

Directions
Mash the avocado. Set aside in a bowl. Put sour cream (or yogurt, if using) in a bowl. Add lime juice, cilantro and ground cumin. Stir until just mixed. Add mashed avocados and stir until well mixed. Carefully place about a spoonful of the avocado mixture into each of the endive leaves. Serve.

Serves: 4	**Prep Time:15 mins.**	**Cooking Time:37 mins.**
Calories: 90	**Protein:4g**	**Carbs:14g**	**Fat:9g**

143. Cannellini Bean Cookies

Ingredients:

1 egg
1 can (14 oz) cannellini beans, drained and rinsed
¼ cup olive oil
½ cup brown sugar

1 cup rolled oats
2 oz chocolate (dark), chopped
½ cup almonds (raw), chopped
½ cup flour (self-raising), whole wheat
1/3 cup ginger (candied), chopped

Directions:

Preheat oven to 350°F (180°C). Oil two baking trays lightly. In a food processor or blender, puree the cannellini beans. Add the sugar, egg, and olive oil. Mix the ingredients until combined well. In a large bowl, combine the almond, oats, ginger, and chocolate. Fold in the bean mixture and stir to combine. Add in the flour and stir briefly. Spoon two tablespoonful of the batter for each cookie. Spoon on to the baking trays and press the dough into flat circles. For 20 minutes, bake the cookies, or until they're browned evenly.

Serves: 24   Prep Time:15 mins.   Cooking Time:20 mins.
Calories:111   Protein:3g   Carbs:12g   Fat:6g

144. Chocolate Brownies

Ingredients:

2 eggs
1 can (15 oz) black beans (drained), rinsed
2 tbsp olive oil
¼ cup cocoa powder, dark
3 ½ oz dark chocolate (melted), slightly cooled

½ cup brown sugar
1 tsp baking powder
1 pinch salt
2 tsp vanilla extract
1 cup pecans, chopped

Directions:

Preheat oven to 350°F (180°C). Grease lightly a square cake tin (20cm). Use parchment paper to line the base, extending over two opposite sides. In a food processor, combine the ingredients, with the exception of the pecans. Process until well combined and smooth. Spread the mixture on to the tin and smoothen out the top surface. Sprinkle over the pecans and press gently into the mixture. Bake the brownie mix for 25 minutes, or until its center is firm yet gentle to the touch. Leave for 5 minutes before removing from baking tin. Transfer the brownies to a wire rack and remove the parchment paper. Cool the brownies completely, before cutting it into 16 smaller squares.

Serves: 16   Prep Time:15 mins.   Cooking Time:25 mins.
Calories:165   Protein:4g   Carbs:13g   Fat:12g

145. MIND Friendly Banana Avocado Chocolate Cookies

Ingredients:

1 banana

1 egg

1 cup avocado flesh, very ripe

½ cup cocoa powder, dark

½ tsp baking soda

Chocolate chunks (dark), to taste

2 tbsp honey (raw), optional

Directions:

Preheat the oven to 350°F. In a bowl, combine the avocado, banana, and honey. Use a hand mixer or transfer to a food processor and mix the ingredients until you get a smooth consistency. Blend in the baking soda, cocoa powder, and egg, and continue to mix until the ingredients are blended well. Add in the dark chocolate chunks. By the spoonful, drop cookie dough on a parchment paper-lined baking sheet. Bake until the cookies are firm and warm, or for 8 to 10 minutes.

Serves: 4	Prep Time:15 mins.		Cooking Time:10 mins.
Calories:339	Protein:6.7g	Carbs:65g	Fat:10.2g

146. Blueberry Ice Cream

Ingredients:

1 cup (150g) blueberries

1 can (14 oz) coconut milk, full-fat

1 tsp rosemary, minced

2 tbsp. honey, raw

2 egg yolks

1 tsp lemon extract

Directions:

In a food processor or blender, combine the blueberries, coconut milk, rosemary, honey, and lemon extract. Blend until you achieve a smooth consistency. In a saucepan on medium-high heat, pour the mixture and add egg yolks. Whisk continually until you bring the mixture to a low boil. As it starts to boil, remove the mixture and cool.

Transfer the blueberry mix into a bowl and cover with cling wrap. Place in the refrigerator for a minimum of 2 hours. You can also refrigerate overnight. Transfer the mix into an ice cream maker and churn until you reach the right consistency. Scoop out the ice cream immediately. You may store in the freezer or serve the ice cream immediately.

Serves: 4	Prep Time:5 mins.		Cooking Time:10 mins.
Calories:358	Protein:4.2g	Carbs:29g	Fat:27.5g

147. *Coconut, Chia, Chocolate Cookies*

Ingredients:

7 oz dates, pitted

½ cup walnuts

½ cup coconut, shredded

2 tbsp cocoa powder, raw

1 tsp vanilla extract

1 tbsp chia seeds

Directions:

Preheat oven to 350° (180°C). On a baking tray, spread out the walnuts and bake until toasted lightly, or for 4 to 5 minutes. Cool the walnuts on a plate, then chop roughly. In a food processor, add the dates, cocoa powder, coconut, vanilla, 1/3 of the walnuts, and chia seeds. Process until the ingredients are combined well. In a bowl, put the rest of the chopping walnuts. Roll a heaped teaspoon of the chocolate mix into a ball. Flatten slightly, then press gently the top into the walnuts. Do the same with the rest of the mixture. Place the cookies in one layer in a container. Chill until the cookies harden. You can refrigerate the cookies for about 2 weeks.

Serves: 24	Prep Time:15 mins.		Cooking Time:5 mins.
Calories:53	Protein:1g	Carbs:6g	Fat:3g

148. *Mixed Berry Pudding*

Ingredients:

2 cups mixed berries, frozen

2 cups buttermilk

1 tbsp maple syrup

2 tbsp confectioner's sugar

1 vanilla bean

1/6 oz gelatin sheets

Directions:

In a small saucepan, mix the sugar and the buttermilk. Split the vanilla lengthwise and scrape the seeds into the saucepan. Add in the bean. Heat the mixture gently until it's hot but not boiling. Turn the heat off and let stand for 10 minutes. Remove the bean. In a bowl of water (cold), soak the gelatin sheets for 5 minutes to soften them. Squeeze the water out. Add the gelatin to the sugar-buttermilk mix and stir until the mixture's dissolved.

Oil lightly 4 dariole molds (1/2 cup). Pour the mixture and chill until set, or for 4 hours. In a saucepan, heat the berries gently until juicy and thawed. Stir the maple syrup into the saucepan. Before serving, invert each dariole mold on to a plate. Hold the plate with your hands and the mold with your thumbs. Shake to dislodge the concoction. Spoon berries over the buttermilk pudding.

Serves: 4	Prep Time:15 mins.		Cooking Time:10 mins.
Calories:169	Protein:7g	Carbs:26g	Fat:3g

149. Cranberry, Ginger, and Pear Crumble

Ingredients:

Fruit:

2 tsp confectioner's sugar

2 lb pears (or 5 large pears)

1 tsp vanilla extract

½ cup cranberries (dried), halved

Crumble Topping:

½ cup ginger, ground

1/3 cup whole wheat flour

½ cup rolled oats

2 oz olive oil spread

2 tbsp brown sugar

2 tbsp shredded coconut

1/3 cup pecans, chopped

Directions:

Preheat oven to 375°F (190°C). Peel the pears. Core and quarter them. Chop them up roughly and put in a large saucepan. Sprinkle with the confectioner's sugar. Cover the pan and boil. Reduce heat. On medium-low, cook the pears for 5 more minutes. Add in the cranberries. To make the crumble, sift the ginger and flour in a bowl.

Add the olive oil spread. Use fingers until the ingredients are combined evenly. Add in the coconut, oats, pecans, and brown sugar. Sprinkle the crumble topping over the pears in the baking dish. Bake the dish for 30 minutes, or until the topping is golden brown. Serve the crumble warm, with low-fat ice cream or low-fat custard.

Serves: 6   **Prep Time:25 mins.**   **Cooking Time:40 mins.**

Calories:255   **Protein:3.5g**   **Carbs:33.5g**   **Fat:14.5g**

150. *Pistachio and Saffron Pudding*

Ingredients:

Puddings:

3 cups milk, low-fat

½ cup pistachios, raw

1 pinch saffron threads

1 ½ tbsp currants

2 pods cardamom

1 stick cinnamon

1 1/3 fine semolina

1 tsp rosewater

2 tbsp honey

Syrup:

2 pods cardamom, crushed

1 ½ tbsp honey

Directions:

Grind or finely chop half of the pistachios. Chop coarsely the rest of the pistachios and set aside. In a large saucepan, combine the currants, milk, cinnamon stick, cardamom pods, and saffron threads. Let the mixture stand for 1 hour. Boil the mixture. Remove the cinnamon and add in semolina and honey.

Beat the mixture until you get a smooth consistency. Stir in the rosewater and the pistachios (finely chopped). Mix well. Pour or spoon the mixture into 4 (200ml) serving dishes or glasses. For the syrup, mix together the cardamom pods and honey in a saucepan. Bring the mixture to a boil. Top the puddings with honey syrup, hot cardamom, and the rest of the pistachios. Serve and enjoy.

Serves: 4   **Prep Time:20 mins.**   **Cooking Time:15 mins.**

Calories:432   **Protein:18g**   **Carbs:68g**   **Fat:10g**

151. Raspberry and Banana Yogurt Ice Cream

Ingredients:

1 cup Greek yogurt, low-fat

3 bananas (large), ripe

7 oz raspberries, frozen

1 tsp vanilla extract

Slice the bananas into ¾" (2cm) portions and put in a Ziploc bag. Remove the excess air, and seal tightly. Freeze the bananas until firm or for about 6 hours. Meanwhile, use muslin or cheesecloth to line a sieve. Stand over one bowl, with the sieve well bottom clear of the bowl's base. Spoon the yogurt into the cloth. Gather the cloth's ends and twist to close. Put a sauce on top of the cloth and weigh it down with 2 cans (14 oz or 400g).

Refrigerate to drain for around 4 hours. In a food processor, combine the frozen banana, raspberries, yogurt, and vanilla. Blend until evenly combined and smooth in consistency. Stop occasionally and use a rubber spatula to scrape the sides. Place the mixture in a container and freeze until firm or for about 6 hours. Before serving, remove from the freezer for about 10 minutes. If you wish to serve the yogurt individually, freeze the mixture in Popsicle molds.

Serves: 8   **Prep Time:20 mins.**   **Cooking Time: 0 mins.**

Calories:238   **Protein:14g**   **Carbs:34g**   **Fat:5g**

152. Lemon & Blueberry Swirl Bars
Ingredients

2 cups cashew nuts

1/2 cup fresh lemon juice

3/4 cup plus 1 extra tablespoon coconut milk

1/2 cup melted coconut oil

1/4 cup maple syrup

2 teaspoons finely grated lemon rind

1 1/2 teaspoons vanilla extract

3/4 cup frozen blueberries, thawed in a bowl

Base

1 tablespoon coconut oil

1/2 cup lightly toasted sunflower seeds

1/2 cup lightly toasted cashew nuts

1/2 cup lightly toasted desiccated coconut

1 cup pitted fresh dates, chopped

Pinch sea salt

Directions

Put the cashews in a mixing bowl. Pour cold water to fully submerge the cashews. Soak the nuts for 4 hours. After soaking, drain and rinse the nuts under running cold water. Get an 8-inch square pan. Grease the bottom and the sides. Line the pan with baking or parchment paper, with some of the paper overhanging from the sides of the pan. Place cashews (lightly toasted), coconut and sunflower seeds in a food processor. Pulse until everything is coarsely chopped. Add salt, oil and dates. Pulse again until the ingredients form an evenly combined mixture. Transfer to the prepared baking pan. Press down to form a smooth, even crust. Chill the crust in the refrigerator until firm, about 30 minutes.

Place the soaked cashews in a food processor or high-speed blender. Add the rind, vanilla, 100 ml of the melted coconut oil, milk, maple syrup and juice. Blend the ingredients with a few pulses until it becomes a smooth mixture. Place 2/3 of this cashew mixture into a mixing bowl. Add the extra tablespoon of coconut milk. Stir and spoon into the prepared crust. Place the berries into the blender. Add the rest of the melted coconut oil into the blender. Pulse until smooth. Spoon this cashew-berry mixture at random places on the pan. Use a butter knife to create blueberry swirls. Chill until set. Once set, place the pan at room temperature to slightly soften. Once slightly soft, slice into 18 bars.

Serves: 18	Prep Time: 6 hrs.		Cooking Time:0 mins.
Calories:128	Protein:5g	Carbs:14g	Fat:23g

153. Macadamia balls

Ingredients

12 pitted medjool dates

1 teaspoon vanilla extract

1 tablespoon honey

1/2 cup coconut spread

1/2 cup shredded coconut

2/3 cup macadamia meal

1 tablespoon cocoa

1/4 cup roughly chopped dried apricots

Directions

Put ½ cup of the macadamia meal in a food processor. Put in the coconut spread, ¼ cup of coconut, cocoa powder, apricots, vanilla, dates and honey as well. Pulse to combine the ingredients into a thick, smooth, paste-like mixture. In a small bowl, mix the rest of coconut and macadamia meal. Mix and set aside. Transfer the mixture from the food processor into a shallow dish. Scoop out the coconut-macadamia paste by the tablespoon and roll into balls. Roll the balls into the coconut mixture in the small bowl. Arrange the coated balls on a plate. Chill the balls to firm up in the refrigerator. Serve once firm.

Serves: 6	Prep Time:15 mins. + chilling time	Cooking Time:0 mins.
Calories:470	Protein:2.1g Carbs:8g	Fat:8g

154. Chia Sesame Balls

Ingredients

1/3 cup toasted macadamias

1/3 cup dry roasted cashews

1 cup pitted dried dates

1 tablespoon rice malt syrup

2 tablespoons white chia seeds

2 tablespoons sesame seeds, toasted

Directions

Place half of the sesame seeds, macadamia, cashews, chia seeds, dates and rice malt syrup in a blender or food processor. Pulse the ingredients until a well-mixed, paste-like, thick and smooth mixture is formed. Transfer the mixture into a shallow dish. Place the remaining sesame seeds on a plate. Scoop out 2 tablespoons of the nut-seeds mixture. Roll into balls. Coat the balls by rolling on the sesame seeds. Place the coated balls on a plate. Chill to set the balls in the refrigerator. Serve once firm.

Serves: 6	Prep Time:15 mins. + chilling time	Cooking Time:0 mins.
Calories:263	Protein:1.2g Carbs:6.5g	Fat:3.4g

155. Granola

Ingredients

1½ cups walnuts, pecans, or almonds

1/2 cup dried dates (optional)

2 Tbs almond flour

1/3 cup liquid coconut oil

1/4 cup maple syrup

1 tsp vanilla extract

3½ cups rolled oats

1/2 cup pumpkin seeds

1 Tbs hemp seeds

1 tsp pine nuts

1/3 cup chunky salted almond butter

1 tsp cinnamon

1/2 tsp ground nutmeg

1/4 tsp ground cardamom

1 Tbs chia seeds

1/2 cup shredded unsweetened coconut

Directions

Chop nuts and dates. Toss dates with almond flour. In a small bowl, mix liquid ingredients. In a large bowl, mix dry ingredients; stir well. Pour wet ingredients into dry, stirring frequently. Spray rimmed baking sheet with coconut oil, spread granola evenly on sheet. Bake at 275 degrees for one hour, stirring every fifteen minutes. When mixture is cool, transfer to bowl and add chia seeds and shredded coconut. Enjoy granola by itself or with plain goat yogurt or your favorite milk. Excess can be frozen.

Serves: 12	Prep Time: 15 mins.		Cooking Time: 1 hr.
Calories: 453	Protein: 10.23g	Carbs: 80g	Fat: 12.24g

156. Avocado Goji and Chia Pudding

Ingredients

1 cup unsweetened coconut or almond milk

1 avocado

2 tablespoons honey

1 banana

1/3 cup goji berries

3 tablespoons chia seeds

Directions

Puree milk, banana, honey and avocado. When mixture is smooth, stir in goji berries and chia seeds. Pour the pudding mixture into prepared Popsicle molds. Freeze the pops until set, for at least 8 hours.

Serves: 5	Prep Time:15 mins. + freezing time		Cooking Time:0 mins.
Calories:166	Protein:4g	Carbs:21g	Fat:8g

157.   Peanut Butter Power Bars

Ingredients

1/2 cup rolled oats
1/4 cup unsweetened natural peanut butter
1 1/2 cups pitted Medjool dates
1/2 teaspoon sea salt

1 teaspoon vanilla extract
1/2 cup almonds, roughly chopped
1/2 cup dried cherries

Directions

Place parchment on a 9-by-5-inch loaf pan. Set aside. Place the oats in a blender or food processor. Pulse to coarsely chop but not into a powder. Add peanut butter, salt, vanilla and dates. Process to create a mixture that clumps together. Put the dried cherries into the food processor or blender. Process a few times to mix all ingredients well. Place the mixture into a shallow dish. Add the almonds to the mixture. Knead the mixture to mix well. Transfer into the prepared pan. Place parchment paper on top of the mixture. Press to flatten the mixture and spread evenly on the pan. Chill until the mixture sets, about 1 hour or so. Once set, slice into bars.

Serves: 12	**Prep Time: 1 hr. 15 mins.**	**Cooking Time:0 mins.**
Calories:151	**Protein:3g** **Carbs:23g**	**Fat:6g**

158.   Chocolate Zesty Balls

Ingredients

3/4 cup pitted Medjool dates
1 cup almonds or cashews
1/4 cup unsweetened cocoa or raw cacao powder
1 teaspoon vanilla extract

Pinch of salt
2 tablespoons cacao nibs
1 tablespoon grated orange zest
More orange zest or shredded coconut, for dusting

Directions

Put cashews in a blender or food processor. Pulse the cashews until it becomes crumbly. Put vanilla, salt, cacao powder and dates with the crumbly cashews. Process a few times. Put the cacao nibs and orange zest as well. Pulse again a few times. Transfer the mixture to a shallow dish. Scoop out mixture enough for 1-inch balls. Roll. Chill the mixture until firm if it is too wet or sticky to work with. Dust each of the balls with some orange zest or coconut. Arrange the balls on a cookie sheet. Chill the balls for 1 hour then serve once set.

Serves: 20	**Prep Time: 1 hr. 15 mins.**	**Cooking Time:0 mins.**
Calories:82	**Protein:2g** **Carbs:8g**	**Fat:5g**

159. Apple and Mulberry Crisps

Ingredients

Olive oil cooking spray

3/4 cup apple cider

3/4 cup dried mulberries

1 tablespoon fresh lemon juice

6 cups Golden Delicious or Fuji peeled apples

1 1/2 teaspoons ground cinnamon

1/2 teaspoon salt

4 1/2 tablespoons turbinado sugar

3/4 cup old-fashioned rolled oats

2 tablespoons white chia seeds

2 tablespoon all-purpose flour

1/4 cup finely chopped walnuts

1/4 cup cold diced coconut oil

Vanilla yogurt, for serving

Directions

Prepare the oven to 375F. Lightly grease a 7-by-11-inch baking dish using cooking spray. Mix cider and mulberries in a large bowl. Set aside to stand for about 10 minutes. Place cinnamon, ¼ teaspoon salt, 3 tablespoons sugar, lemon juice and apples into the bowl with the mulberry-cider mixture. Get another bowl and mix the remaining ¼ teaspoon salt, 1 ½ tablespoons sugar, chia seeds, flour and oats. Add the coconut oil and cut it into the mixture using a pastry blender or 2 knives. Work the coconut oil in until the mixture looks like coarse sand. Stir the walnuts in. Transfer the apple mixture into the prepared pan. Flatten into an even layer. Spread the oat mixture over the apple mixture layer. Bake into the preheated oven until it becomes bubbly and golden brown. This takes around 30 to 35 minutes. Remove from the oven and slightly cool. Serve topped with a scoop of yogurt.

Serves: 8	Prep Time:15 mins.		Cooking Time:45 mins.
Calories:115	Protein:4g	Carbs:40g	Fat:10g

160. Energy Bars

Ingredients

1/2 cup dried dates

2 cups raw almonds

1/2 cup maple syrup

2/3 cup coconut oil

2 tsp vanilla

1 tsp Himalayan salt

1/2 cup sunflower seeds

1 tsp cinnamon

1/2 tsp nutmeg

4 cups oats

1 cup shredded coconut

3/4 cup sliced almonds

1/4 cup chia seeds

1/3 cup dark chocolate chips

Directions

Chop dates; be careful of the pits! Line a 9" x 9" baking pan with wax paper. In a blender or food processor, combine 2 cups raw almonds, maple syrup, coconut oil, vanilla, and salt. In a separate bowl, combine remaining ingredients. Stir in almond mixture. Spread into pan and press evenly. Let sit at room temperature 8–12 hours or overnight. Cut into bars.

Serves: 8	Prep Time:15 mins. + 12 hr. setting time		Cooking Time:0 mins.
Calories: 250	Protein: 10g	Carbs: 44g	Fat: 5g

161. Cappuccino Superfood Panna Cota

Ingredients

1 13.5-oz. can coconut milk
1 teaspoon instant espresso granules
1/3 cup turbinado sugar
1/8 teaspoon salt
1/4 teaspoon ground cinnamon

1 cup whole-milk plain kefir
1 1/4-oz. pack unflavored gelatin
1 teaspoon vanilla extract
Dark chocolate curls, as garnish

Directions

Put milk into a large, deep cup. Whisk well. Pour 1 cup of the whisked milk into a medium-sized pan. Add salt, cinnamon, espresso and sugar. Whisk to mix. Sprinkle gelatin powder over the milk mixture. Set aside to stand for about 5 minutes. Put the pan with the milk-gelatin mixture over a stove on medium heat setting. Cook the mixture. Stir constantly for 1 to 2 minutes until it turns smooth.

Get another bowl. Whisk the remaining ¾ cup of milk with vanilla and kefir. Slowly pour the gelatin mixture into the milk-kefir mixture, constantly whisking while adding. Divide and pour the mixture between 6 ramekins. Chill to set the panna cotta. Once firm, serve with a garnish of chocolate curls.

Serves: 6	Prep Time: 15 mins. + chilling time	Cooking Time:0 mins.
Calories:115	Protein: 4g	Carbs:17g	Fat:16g

162. Smoothie Peach Pie Bowl

Ingredients

1 1/2 cups frozen peaches
3/4 cup non-fat plain Greek yogurt
1/2 cup milk
1 tablespoon almond butter
1 tablespoon honey
1/2 teaspoon cinnamon

1/2 teaspoon vanilla extract
pinch of nutmeg
Toppings:
granola
fresh peach slices
toasted sliced almond

Directions

Place all the main ingredients a blender. Pulse into a smooth and creamy blend. Pour into a serving bowl. Neatly arrange the toppings on top of the smoothie. Serve immediately.

Serves: 6	Prep Time:15 mins.	Cooking Time:0 mins.
Calories:358	Protein:22.2g	Carbs:40g	Fat:14.5g

163. Superfood Pudding

Ingredients

1/2 cup sliced almonds
1 can coconut milk
2 cups plain Greek yogurt
3 Tbs plus 6 tsp maple syrup

1/2 cup chia seeds
2 tsp vanilla
1/2 tsp Himalayan salt
2 pints blueberries

Directions

Toast almonds in a dry skillet over medium heat, stirring frequently; remove from heat and allow to cool. Mix the coconut milk, Greek yogurt, 3 tablespoons maple syrup, chia, vanilla, and Himalayan salt. Cover and refrigerate for eight to twelve hours, stirring occasionally. Mix the blueberries with the remaining 6 teaspoons maple syrup. Stir in almonds. Serve in dishes with alternating layers of chia mixture and berries.

Serves: 6	Prep Time:15 mins.		Cooking Time:0 mins.
Calories:69	Protein:3.1g	Carbs:7.5g	Fat:2.8g

164. Chocolate Date Balls

Ingredients

2 Tbs pine nuts
1 cup shredded coconut
2 cups dates
2 cups almond meal
1/2 cup almond butter
1 Tbs chia seeds

1 tsp cinnamon
1 cup unsweetened cocoa powder
1/4 cup maple syrup
1/4 cup water
Additional ground nuts or coconut flakes for rolling, optional

Directions

If you wish to, toast the pine nuts or coconut in a dry skillet over medium-high heat, stirring constantly until toasted. Chop dates (being careful of the pits), and dust with almond meal. Mix with the other ingredients in a large bowl. You will probably want to use your hands or a food processor to mix well, as the batter can be hard to stir. Use additional water or almond meal to improve the texture if necessary. Form into 1-inch balls, and roll in the ground nuts or coconut flakes if desired. Freeze at least one hour before serving.

Serves: 24	Prep Time:10 mins. + freezing time		Cooking Time:0 mins.
Calories: 65.5	Protein: 1.2g	Carbs: 14.9g	Fat: 1.3g

Mind Diet Smoothies

165. Strawberry Pomegranate Smoothie

Ingredients:

¾ cup strawberries (unsweetened), frozen

2 tsp honey, raw

1/3 cup pomegranate juice

1 tbsp flaxseed oil

1 tbsp yogurt (plain), fat-free

4 ice cubes

Directions:

Whisk the honey and pomegranate juice in a small cup. Completely dissolve the honey. In a blender, combine the yogurt, strawberries, flaxseed oil, pomegranate mixture, and ice cubes. Blend for 1 to 2 minutes, or until smooth and thick. Pour the blended mixture in a glass. Serve and enjoy.

Serves: 1   **Prep Time:8 mins.**   **Cooking Time: 0 mins.**

Calories:262   **Protein:3g**   **Carbs:35g**   **Fat:14g**

166. Blueberry Green Tea Smoothie

Ingredients:

1 bag green tea

3 tbsp water

1 ½ cups blueberries, frozen

2 tsp honey, raw

½ banana, medium

¾ cup vanilla-flavored soy milk, light and calcium-fortified

Directions:

On high, microwave the water until it's hot and steaming. Place the tea bag in it and let it steep for 3 minutes. Remove the bag. Stir in the honey to the tea until it's thoroughly dissolved. In a blender, blend all the ingredients on high until smooth. Serve and enjoy.

Serves: 2   **Prep Time:7 mins.**   **Cooking Time: 0 mins.**

Calories:125   **Protein:1.8g**   **Carbs:29g**   **Fat:1.3g**

167. Beet-Almond-Blueberry Smoothie

Ingredients:

½ cup raw beet, peeled and grated
½ cup blueberries, fresh or frozen
½ cup carrot juice, unsweetened
½ cup applesauce, unsweetened

½ cup raw almonds (whole), unsalted
½ tsp lime juice, fresh
½ cup ice cubes
Dash of ginger, ground

Directions:

Place all the ingredients in a blender. Puree until creamy and smooth. Serve immediately and enjoy.

Serves: 1	Prep Time:5 mins.		Cooking Time: 0 mins.
Calories:325	Protein:10g	Carbs:35g	Fat:18.9g

168. Almond-Banana-Blueberry Smoothie

Ingredients:

¾ of a frozen banana, medium
1 ½ cups almond milk, unsweetened and plain
1 cup kale, chopped

1 cup blueberries, fresh or frozen
2 tsp honey, raw
5 whole almonds, unsalted

Directions:

Place all the ingredients in a blender. Puree for 1 to 2 minutes, or until smooth.

Serves: 1	Prep Time:5 mins.		Cooking Time: 0 mins.
Calories:323	Protein:7g	Carbs:60g	Fat:9.7g

169. Almond Smoothie

Ingredients:

¾ cup almond milk
1 small sliced banana, frozen
¾ cup kale, stems removed and slightly packed

¾ tbsp almond butter
1/8 tsp nutmeg
1/8 tsp cinnamon
1/8 tsp ginger, ground

Directions:

Place all the ingredients in a blender. Blend them until smooth. Serve and enjoy.

Serves: 1	Prep Time:5 mins.		Cooking Time: 0 mins.
Calories:236	Protein:5.4g	Carbs:37g	Fat:9.7g

170. Anti-Inflammatory Smoothie

Ingredients:

½ cup raspberries
½ cup blueberries
¼ cup pineapple, diced
½ banana (small), peeled and frozen
2 tbsp chia seeds

½ cup pomegranate juice
3 ice cubes
1 serving vanilla-flavored whey protein
powder

Directions:

Except for the whey powder, place all the ingredients in a blender. At high speed, blend until smooth. Add in the protein powder, and blend slightly until incorporated.

Serves: 1	Prep Time:5 mins.		Cooking Time: 0 mins.
Calories:380	Protein:24g	Carbs:67g	Fat:4.4g

171. Avocado-Mango Smoothie

Ingredients:

1 cup spinach, fresh
½ mango, fresh
¼ avocado

1 cup vanilla soymilk (low-fat), chilled
5 tsp agave nectar

Directions:

Place all the ingredients in the blender. Puree for 1 to 2 minutes, or until smooth. Serve and enjoy.

Serves: 1	Prep Time:5 mins.		Cooking Time: 0 mins.
Calories:304	Protein:8g	Carbs:57g	Fat:7.5g

172. Spinach Smoothie

Ingredients

2 cups water
2 cups spinach
1 cup lettuce
1 apple

1 pear
1 banana
2 tablespoon fresh lemon juice

Directions

Wash the apple and pear carefully and peel them. Chop the fruits roughly. Combine the chopped fruits, spinach, and lettuce in the blender and start to blend it for 30 seconds. Then peel the banana and chop it. Add the chopped banana in the blender and continue to blend the mass for 2 minutes or till you get smooth mass. Then add lemon juice and blend the smoothie for 20 seconds more. Enjoy!

Serves: 4	Prep Time:15 mins.		Cooking Time:0 mins.
Calories:83	Protein:1.2g	Carbs:20.8g	Fat:0.4g

173. Coconut Citrus Smoothie

Ingredients:

1 cup coconut water

2 tablespoons coconut milk

2 cups of citrus fruit - oranges, grapefruit, lime

1 teaspoon ground turmeric

1/4 teaspoon vanilla extract

1 teaspoon honey

1/4 cup unsweetened rolled oats

1/2 cup ice cubes

Directions:

Place the fiber-filled oats in a blender and grind until they are broken down into a consistency that is close to powder. Add the remaining ingredients and blend until everything is combined and you have the consistency you like in a smoothie. You can omit the ice if you prefer to drink it at room temperature. Pour into a glass and enjoy.

When you incorporate turmeric recipes into your daily diet, you'll be gaining a number of health benefits. The anti-oxidants found in the spice will ensure your body is able to fight off diseases and illnesses. You'll have an easier time digesting your food, and you'll also protect your joints from arthritis. In addition to the health benefits, you'll be able to enjoy spicy, delicious foods that leave you satisfied.

Serves: 1	Prep Time:10 mins.		Cooking Time:26 mins.
Calories:230	Protein:11.6g	Carbs:95.9g	Fat:12.5g

174. Cilantro Smoothie

Ingredients

2 cups cilantro

1 cup parsley

1 teaspoon ginger

2 cups water

1 green apple

1 teaspoon lemon juice

Directions

Wash the cilantro and parsley and chop them roughly. Chop the apple. Combine the chopped cilantro, parsley, apple, and the ginger in the blender and blend the mass for 1 minute. After this, add water and continue to blend the smoothie for 2 minutes more. Then add the lemon juice and blend the mass for 20 seconds more. Ladle the smoothie into the glasses and serve it immediately. Enjoy!

Serves: 2	Prep Time:13 mins.		Cooking Time:0 mins.
Calories:76	Protein:1.6g	Carbs:18.6g	Fat:0.6g

175. *Lime Smoothie*
Ingredients

3 tablespoon lime juice   1 banana
1 teaspoon lemon zest   ½ cup watercress
1 cucumber   1 cup water

Directions
Wash the cucumber and chop it. Combine the watercress and the chopped cucumber together in the blender. Add the banana, lemon zest, and water. Start to blend the mixture for 3 minutes. You should get the smooth and homogeneous mass. Then add the lime juice and blend the mixture for 10 seconds more. Ladle the smoothie into the glasses and serve it immediately. Enjoy!

Serves: 2	Prep Time:13 mins.		Cooking Time:0 mins.
Calories:77	Protein:1.9g	Carbs:19.2g	Fat:0.4g

176. *Apple detox smoothie*
Ingredients
1/3 cup walnuts   1 cup water
2 green apples   ½ cup ice cubes
1 cup parsley   1 banana

Directions
Crush the walnuts gently and transfer them to the food processor. Then peel apples and the banana and chop them roughly. Place the chopped apples and the banana in the food processor too. Add water and start to blend the mixture for 3 minutes. Then add ice cubes and continue to blend it for 1 minute more. Then remove the smoothie from the food processor and ladle it into the glasses. Enjoy!

Serves: 3	Prep Time:13 mins.		Cooking Time:0 mins.
Calories:205	Protein:4.8g	Carbs:32.2g	Fat:8.8g

177. Basil Smoothie

Ingredients

2 cups green basil

½ cup dill

1 tablespoon fresh parsley root

1 lemon

1 cups water

1 tablespoon grapefruit juice

Directions

Place all the ingredients except the lemon in the food processor and start to blend the mixture for 1 minute. Peel the lemon and chop it roughly. Add the chopped lemon in the food processor and continue to blend the smoothie for 1 minute more. Then remove the smoothie from the blender and ladle it into the glasses. Enjoy!

Serves: 2   **Prep Time:12 mins.**   **Cooking Time:0 mins.**

Calories:47   **Protein:3.6g**   **Carbs:10.7g**   **Fat:0.8g**

178. Sweet Green Smoothie

Ingredients

1 avocado

1 cup spinach

1 tablespoon fresh ginger

1 banana

1 kiwi

½ cup water

Directions

Peel the avocado, kiwi, and banana. Chop the ingredients roughly. Place the all the ingredients from the list below in the blender and blend the mixture for 2 minutes. When you get smooth and homogenous mass – ladle the smoothie into the glasses and serve it immediately or keep the smoothie in the fridge.

Serves: 4   **Prep Time:12 mins.**   **Cooking Time:0 mins.**

Calories:294   **Protein:3.7g**   **Carbs:30.1g**   **Fat:20.2g**

179. *Lettuce Smoothie*
Ingredients
1 cup lettuce

½ cup sunflower sprouts

1 carrot

1 banana

1 teaspoon ginger

2 tablespoon lemon juice

Directions
Place the lettuce, sunflower sprouts, and the ginger in the food processor. Peel the carrot and banana and chop them roughly. Add the chopped carrot in the food processor too and start to blend the mixture for 1 minute. Pour the lemon juice into the smoothie and continue to blend it for 20 seconds more. Ladle the smoothie into the serving glasses and serve them immediately.

Serves: 1   Prep Time:15 mins.   Cooking Time:0 mins.

Calories:151   Protein:2.4g   Carbs:36.5g   Fat:0.8g

180. *Green Tea Smoothie*
Ingredients
2 cups green tea

3 handfuls romaine

1 kiwi, peeled

1 cup grapes

1/3 cup cilantro

1 tablespoon lemon juice

1.2 teaspoon raw maca

Directions
Place the grapes, kiwi, romaine, and cilantro in the blender and start to blend the mixture for 2 minutes. Then add raw maca, green tea, and lemon juice and continue to blend the mass for 20 seconds more. When you get smooth and homogenous mass – remove the smoothie from the blender and serve it immediately.

Serves: 1   Prep Time:15 mins.   Cooking Time:0 mins.

Calories:116   Protein:1.9g   Carbs:28g   Fat:0.9g

181. Watercress Smoothie

Ingredients

3 cups watercress

1 cup pineapple

1 orange

½ cup parsley

1 teaspoon lemon juice

Directions

Peel the orange and chop it roughly. Place the watercress, pineapple, chopped orange, parsley, and the lemon juice in the blender and start to blend the mixture on the low speed for 30 seconds. Then increase the speed of the blender till you get maximum speed and blend the smoothie for 1 minute more. Ladle the smoothie into the serving glasses or jar and serve it. Enjoy!

Serves: 1   Prep Time:15 mins.   Cooking Time:0 mins.

Calories:101   Protein:3.3g   Carbs:22.8g   Fat:0.6g

182. Kale Smoothie

Ingredients

1 cups kale

1 cup yerba mate

1 kiwi, peeled

1 pear

½ teaspoon raw cacao

1 teaspoon lemon juice

¼ cup parsley

1 teaspoon fresh ginger

Directions

Chop the pear and kiwi roughly and transfer them to the food processor. Add kale, raw cacao, parsley, and the fresh ginger. Start to blend the mixture on the low speed for 1 minute. Then add the lemon juice and yerba mate. Increase the food processor speed till maximum and blend the mass for 1 minute more. When you get smooth and homogenous mass – remove the smoothie from the food processor and serve it immediately. Enjoy!

Serves: 1   Prep Time:15 mins.   Cooking Time:0 mins.

Calories:173   Protein:4g   Carbs:41.6g   Fat:0.9g

183. Soft Banana Smoothie
Ingredients

2 bananas

1/3 cup Greek yogurt

1 ½ tablespoon honey

1 tablespoon fresh ginger

1/3 teaspoon cinnamon

Directions

Peel the banana and chop it roughly. Then peel the fresh ginger and grate it. Place the chopped banana, grated ginger, honey, Greek yogurt, and cinnamon in the blender. Blend the mixture for 2 minutes or till you get smooth mass. Enjoy!

Serves: 2   Prep Time:12 mins.   Cooking Time:0 mins.

Calories:201   Protein:6.6g   Carbs:44.2g   Fat:1.6g

184. Creamy Orange Smoothie
Ingredients

1 orange

1/3 cup fat-free yogurt

3 tablespoon fresh orange juice

1/3 teaspoon mint extract

Directions

Peel the orange and chop it coarsely. Place the chopped orange, fat-free yogurt, orange juice, and mint extract in the food processor and start to mix the mixture on the low speed for 30 seconds. Then reduce the speed to maximum level and mix it for 1 minute more. Serve it!

Serves: 2   Prep Time:10 mins.   Cooking Time:0 mins.

Calories:77   Protein:3.4g   Carbs:16.4g   Fat:0.2g

185. Aromatic Green Tea Smoothie
Ingredients

¼ cup ice cubes

4 tablespoons water

1 cup warm green tea, brewed

3 tablespoons honey

1 teaspoon vanilla extract

1 small banana

¾ cup almond milk

Directions

Combine the brewed green tea with the honey and stir it carefully till honey is dissolved. Then peel the banana and chop it. Place all the ingredients that were listed above in the blender and start to blend the mixture on the low speed. Then increase the speed slowly till you get maximum level. Blend the smoothie for 2 minutes. Then remove the smoothie from the blender and ladle it into the glasses. Serve it immediately and enjoy!

Serves: 2   Prep Time:12 mins.   Cooking Time:0 mins.

Calories:354   Protein:2.7g   Carbs:42.8g   Fat:21.6g

186.   Watermelon Smoothie

Ingredients

13 oz watermelon

1 cup ice cubes

3 tablespoons water

1 teaspoon honey

1 teaspoon fresh mint

1 tablespoon orange juice

Directions

Chop the fresh mint carefully. Combine water with honey and stir the mixture till you get homogenous mass. Then place the ice cubes, watermelon, honey mixture, orange juice, and chopped fresh mint in the blender and start to blend the mass. Continue to blend the smoothie for 1 minute or till you get smooth mass. Then remove the smoothie from the blender and ladle it into the glasses or keep it in the fridge. Enjoy!

Serves: 3   Prep Time:11 mins.   Cooking Time:0 mins.

Calories:47   Protein:0.8g   Carbs:11.7g   Fat:0.2g

187.   Raspberry Smoothie

Ingredients

2 cups unsweetened raspberries

1 cup frozen strawberries

1 teaspoon fresh ginger, grated

1 tablespoon lemon juice

1 tablespoon honey

1 cup soy milk

Directions

Place the unsweetened raspberries and strawberries in the blender and start to blend it for 1 minute. After this, add honey and grated ginger. Continue to blend the mass for 30 seconds more. Then add soy milk and lemon juice. Blend the mixture for 1 minutes more or till you get smooth mass. Serve it immediately. Add the ice cubes if desired.

Serves: 2   Prep Time:13 mins.   Cooking Time:0 mins.

Calories:128   Protein:4.2g   Carbs:23.7g   Fat:2.2g

188.   Tropical Smoothie

Ingredients

1 cup papaya

½ cup pineapple

1 cup fat-free yogurt

½ teaspoon vanilla extract

½ tablespoon honey

1 tablespoon ground flaxseeds

1 cup ice cubes

Directions

Place the papaya, pineapple, honey, and ground flax seeds in the food processor and mix the mixture for 1 minutes. Then add fat-free yogurt and ice cubes. Mix the mixture for 1 minute. Remove the smoothie from the food processor and ladle it into the glasses. Serve it immediately.

Serves: 3   Prep Time:12 mins.   Cooking Time:0 mins.

Calories:105   Protein:5.5g   Carbs:18.8g   Fat:1g

189. Kiwi-soy Smoothie

Ingredients

3 kiwis

1 banana

1 cup soy milk

1 tablespoon honey

1 teaspoon vanilla extract

Directions

Peel the kiwis and banana and chop them. Place the fruits in the blender and add honey and soy milk. Start to blend the mixture for 30 seconds. Then add vanilla extract and continue to blend the smoothie for 1 minute more. Then remove the dish from the blender and ladle it into the glasses. Enjoy!

Serves: 2   **Prep Time:12 mins.**   **Cooking Time:0 mins.**

Calories:226   **Protein:6g**   **Carbs:46.8g**   **Fat:2.9g**

190. Grapefruit Smoothie

Ingredients

1 grapefruit

2 tablespoon honey

1 teaspoon lemon juice

1 cup cherries, pitted

3 tablespoon water

Directions

Peel the grapefruit and chop it coarsely. Combine the lemon juice and honey together and stir the mixture until honey is dissolved. After this, place the cherries, water mixture, grapefruit, and lemon juice in the blender and blend the mixture for 3 minutes on the medium speed. Remove the smoothie from the blender when you get smooth and homogeneous mass. Transfer the smoothie in the serving glasses and serve it immediately. Enjoy!

Serves: 2   **Prep Time:13 mins.**   **Cooking Time:0 mins.**

Calories:229   **Protein:0.9g**   **Carbs:57.5g**   **Fat:0.2g**

191. Mint Smoothie

Ingredients

1 cup fresh mint

1 lime

2 cups green tea, brewed

Directions

Peel the lime and chop it roughly. Chop the fresh mint. Place the chopped fresh mint and lime in the blender and pour the green tea in it. Start to blend the mixture on the low level and then increase the speed till you get maximum level. When you get smooth and homogenous mass – remove the smoothie from the blender and ladle it into the serving glasses. You can add ice cubes if desired. Enjoy!

Serves: 1   **Prep Time:15 mins.**   **Cooking Time:0 mins.**

Calories:60   **Protein:3.5g**   **Carbs:2g**   **Fat:0.8g**

192. Lemon Sweet Smoothie

Ingredients

1 banana

1 lemon

1 teaspoon cinnamon

3 tablespoons honey

3 tablespoons water

1 teaspoon ginger, grated

Directions

Peel the banana and lemon and chop the fruits roughly. Then take the shallow bowl and combine water and honey in it. Stir the mixture carefully till honey is dissolved. Add grated fresh ginger and stir the mixture carefully again. After this, transfer all the ingredients in the blender and sprinkle the mixture with the cinnamon. Blend the mixture for 3 minutes till you get homogenous mass. Then remove the smoothie from the blender and add 1 teaspoon of stevia if it is not sweet enough. Stir it little and serve it. Enjoy!

Serves: 1	Prep Time:15 mins.		Cooking Time:0 mins.
Calories:325	Protein:2.4g	Carbs:87.4g	Fat:0.7g

193. Nutritious Brain Smoothie

Ingredients

3 kiwis

2 bananas

1 cup almond milk

1 teaspoon flaxseeds, ground

1 teaspoon chia seeds

1 tablespoon walnuts

Directions

Crush the walnuts and combine them with the chia seeds and flaxseeds. Transfer the mixture to the blender and add almond milk. Peel the kiwis and the bananas and chop them. Transfer the chopped fruits in the blender too and start to blend the mass on the low speed for 30 seconds. Then increase the speed to maximum level and blend the mixture for 1 minute more. Remove the smoothie from the blender and ladle it into the serving glasses. Enjoy!

Serves: 3	Prep Time:12 mins.		Cooking Time:0 mins.
Calories:321	Protein:4.3g	Carbs:34g	Fat:21.5g

194. Avocado Smoothie

Ingredients

1 avocado

1 cup water

1 banana

1 teaspoon honey

1 scoop vanilla whey protein powder

½ cup strawberries

Directions

Peel the avocado and banana. Chop the vegetables and transfer them to the food processor. Add strawberries and honey and start to blend the mass for 30 seconds. Then add water and vanilla whey protein powder. Blend the mixture for 1 minute more on the high speed. Then remove the smoothie from the blender and ladle it into the glasses. Serve it immediately.

| Serves: 3 | Prep Time:12 mins. | | Cooking Time:0 mins. |
| Calories:225 | Protein:9.2g | Carbs:19.8g | Fat:13.9g |

195. Protein Smoothie

Ingredients

4 envelope Gelatin powder

2 ½ cup coconut milk

2 egg yolks

1 teaspoon vanilla extract

½ cup ice cubes

1 banana

1 teaspoon honey

Directions

Peel the banana and chop it. Place all the ingredients from the list above in the food processor and start to blend the mixture on the low speed for 1 minute. Then increase the speed to the highest level and blend the mass for 30 seconds more. Ladle the smoothie into the serving glasses and add ice cubes if desired. Serve it immediately and enjoy!

| Serves: 4 | Prep Time:15 mins. | | Cooking Time:0 mins. |
| Calories:430 | Protein:11.1g | Carbs:16.9g | Fat:38.1g |

196. Broccoli Brain Boost Smoothie

Ingredients

1 cup broccoli

¼ cup walnuts

1 cup almond milk

3 tablespoon water

1 teaspoon turmeric

1 teaspoon ginger, grated

Directions

Chop the broccoli roughly and transfer it to the blender. Crush the walnuts and combine the nuts with the chopped broccoli. After this, transfer the mixture to the blender and start to blend it for 30 seconds. Then add almond milk, water, turmeric, and grated ginger. Blend the mass for 2 minutes, when you get smooth and homogenous mass – remove it from the blender and ladle it into the glasses. Serve it immediately or keep the smoothie in the fridge not more than 1 day. Enjoy!

Serves: 2	Prep Time:13 mins.		Cooking Time:0 mins.
Calories:395	Protein:7.9g	Carbs:12.5g	Fat:38.1g

197. Delicious Chocolate Smoothie

Ingredients

2 bananas

1 cup Greek yogurt

1 tablespoon almond milk

1 tablespoon cocoa

1 teaspoon honey

1 teaspoon cinnamon

1/3 cup papaya

Directions

Peel the bananas and chop them. Take the shallow bowl and combine cocoa, honey, and cinnamon it. Stir it gently and transfer to the blender. Add chopped bananas and papaya. Then pour Greek yogurt and almond milk into the mixture. Blend the mass for 2 minutes till you get smooth mass. Serve it immediately and enjoy!

Serves: 2	Prep Time:15 mins.		Cooking Time:0 mins.
Calories:228	Protein:12.2g	Carbs:39.3g	Fat:4.6g

198. Nourishing Smoothie

Ingredients

2 ripe bananas

1/2 can (7 oz.) coconut milk or milk of your choice

1 cup plain kefir (easily digestible) or plain yogurt

2 Tbs almond butter

1 Tbs ground flaxseed

1 cup fresh or frozen berries (blueberries and/or raspberries recommended)

2 cups ice

Directions

Combine all ingredients in blender, and blend until smooth. For a little extra flavor, add a few drops of vanilla extract. If desired, add honey to sweeten.

Serves: 2	Prep Time:10 mins.		Cooking Time:0 mins.
Calories: 381	Protein: 15g	Carbs: 81g	Fat: 3g

199. Kid's Smoothie

Ingredients

1/3 cup walnuts, crushed

¾ cup almonds, crushed

2 cups milk

1 banana, peeled

1 cup blueberry

1 tablespoon honey

1 teaspoon stevia extract

Directions

Place all the ingredients that were listed above in the blender and start to blend the mixture on the low speed for 1 minute. Then increase the speed to the maximum level and blend the mixture for 1 minute more. Remove the mixture from the blender and ladle it in the serving glasses. Serve the smoothie immediately. Enjoy!

Serves: 4	Prep Time:15 mins.		Cooking Time:0 mins.
Calories:291	Protein:10.9g	Carbs:27.2g	Fat:17.8g

200. Green Apple Smoothie

Ingredients

1 teaspoon chia seeds

2 green apples, peeled

1 teaspoon cinnamon

1 grapefruit

1 tablespoon honey

1 teaspoon lemon juice

1 tablespoon coconut

1 teaspoon vanilla extract

Directions

Combine lemon juice and honey together and stir it carefully till honey is dissolved. After this, chop the apples roughly. Peel the grapefruit and chop it too. Transfer all the ingredients from the list above in the food processor and blend the mixture for 2 minutes. When you get smooth and homogenous mass – ladle the smoothie into the glasses and serve it. Add ice cubes if deserved. Enjoy!

Serves: 1   **Prep Time:15 mins.**   **Cooking Time:0 mins.**

Calories:374   **Protein:2.4g**   **Carbs:92.5g**   **Fat:2.7g**

201. Carrot Smoothie

Ingredients

2 carrots

1 cup parsley

1 cucumber

1/3 cup water

1 teaspoon dry ginger

2 tablespoon lemon juice

Directions

Peel the carrots and chop it. Chop the parsley and cucumber. Transfer the vegetables to the blender and add water, dry ginger, and lemon juice. Start to blend the mass on the low speed for 1 minute. Then increase the blender speed until maximum and blend the smoothie for 2 minutes more. Ladle the smoothie into the glasses. Serve it immediately.

Serves: 3   **Prep Time:15 mins.**   **Cooking Time:0 mins.**

Calories:43   **Protein:1.7g**   **Carbs:9.5g**   **Fat:0.4g**

202. Super Brain Boosted Smoothie

Ingredients

1 cup milk

1 scoop magnesium beverage powder

1 cup blueberries, frozen

1 banana, peeled, frozen

Directions

Place all the ingredients that were listed above in the blender. Blend the mixture for 3 minutes till you get smooth and homogeneous mass. Then remove the smoothie from the blender and ladle it into the glasses. Serve it immediately. Enjoy!

Serves: 2 **Prep Time:15 mins.** **Cooking Time:0 mins.**

Calories:155 **Protein:5.2g** **Carbs:30g** **Fat:2.9g**

203. Beetroot Smoothie

Ingredients

1 cup beetroot, chopped

1 cup fresh celery

1 carrot

2 tablespoon lemon juice

½ cup sour cream

3 tablespoon water

¼ cup almonds, crushed

Directions

Chop the parsley and transfer it to the blender. Add beetroot, lemon, sour cream, water, and the crushed almonds. Start to blend the mixture for 1 minutes. Then peel the carrot and grate it. Add the grated carrot in the blender and continue to blend the mass for 1 minute more on the high speed. Transfer the smoothie in the glasses. Serve it immediately. Enjoy!

Serves: 2 **Prep Time:15 mins.** **Cooking Time:0 mins.**

Calories:253 **Protein:6.5g** **Carbs:18.3g** **Fat:18.4g**

Conclusion

Thank you for sticking with us all the way to the end! We hope we were able to set you on the right path to selecting and preparing a delicious meal with to help with cognitive functions whether it be for you, a relative or a close friend.

So, what happens next?

Keep practicing and explore new and exciting meals from the MIND diet. Mix and match the delicious recipes presented in this book to come up with your favorite MIND diet meals then share them with your friends, and family!

Once again, thank you for allowing us to help you on this MIND diet journey, and feel free to leave us a positive review if you like what you read through.

Until next time … best of luck!

Made in the USA
Columbia, SC
15 November 2018